Ultimate Guide
for
Type 2 Diabetes Reversal
Deluxe Edition
Bonus: Delicious Simple Recipes

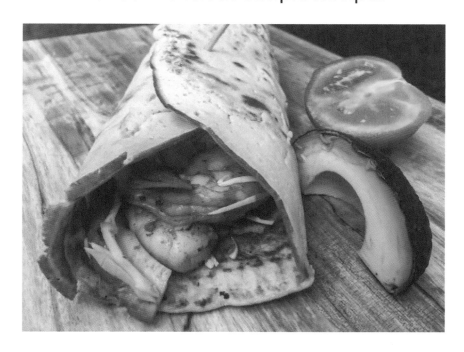

Mimi Chan, RD, LD, CNSC, CDE
Cheng Ruan, MD

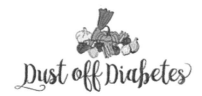

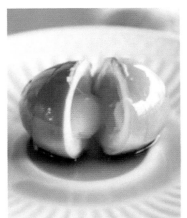
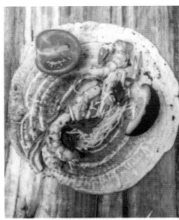
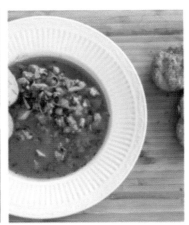
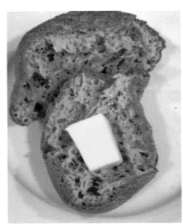

Ultimate Guide for Type 2 Diabetes Reversal

Deluxe Edition

Bonus: Delicious Simple Recipes

Mimi Chan, RD, LD, CNSC, CDE

Cheng Ruan, MD

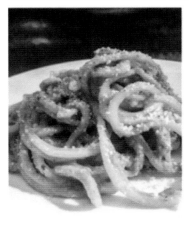
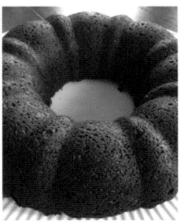
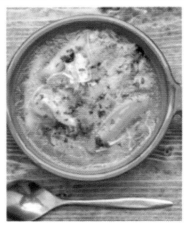
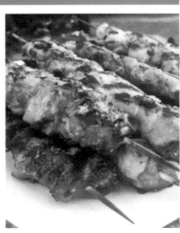

Ultimate Guide for Type 2 Diabetes Reversal Deluxe Edition

Copyright © 2016 Dust Off Diabetes, LLC

Ultimate Guide for Type 2 Diabetes Reversal Deluxe Edition - Bonus: Delicious Simple Recipes is intended solely for informational and educational purposes and is not intended to be a substitute for qualified medical advice. Always seek the advice and counsel of your personal physician with any questions you have regarding a medical condition, and before undertaking any diet, exercise, or other health program.

The authors and publisher specifically disclaim all responsibility for any liability, loss or risk, personal or otherwise, that is incurred as a consequence, directly or indirectly, of the use and application of the contents of this book.

Authors:
Mimi Chan, RD, LD, CNSC, CDE
Cheng Ruan, MD

Published by Dust Off Diabetes, LLC

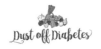
Dust off Diabetes

Table of Contents

Meet Mimi Chan   7
Meet Dr. Cheng Ruan   8
Introduction   9
The Human Psyche (First step in Diabetes reversal)   13
Why the Layers of Living Success (LOLS)   16
Creation of Layer of Living Success   22
Disclaimer   34
Layers of Living Success (LOLS)   35
How to Use LOLS Plan   36
What is LOLS   38
Sample Plates based on Blood Sugar   39
Layer 1: No Daily Limit   41
Layer 2: Preferred Proteins   42
Layer 3: Favorite Fats   43
Layer 4: Low Glycemic Index   44
Layer 5: Preferred Carbohydrates   45
Layer 6: Sparing the Spare Tire   46
Low Blood Sugar Management   47
How to Use Layers Log   48
Layers Log   49

Soups
Hearty Vegetable Soup   54
Kale and White Bean Soup   55
Mulligatawny Soup   56
Hearty Beef Stew   57
Chinese watercress with Pork   58
Lemon Chicken Low Carb Noodle Soup   59
Mexican Chicken Soup with Avocado   60
Chicken Vegetable Soup   61
Japanese Inspired Onion Soup   61
Low Carb Thai Shrimp Soup   62
Tuscan White Bean Soup   63
Low Carb Thai Chicken Zoodle Soup   64
Creamy Zucchini Soup   65
Paleo Seafood Chowder   66
Beef and Onion Soup   67
Sweet Potato Cauliflower Sausage Soup   68

Eggs, Eggs and more Eggs
Simple Scrambled Eggs   70
Perfect Hard Boiled Eggs   71
Perfect Hard Soft Eggs   72
Taragon Soft Scrambled Eggs   73
Shoyu Tamgo (Soy Sauce Egg)   74
Crust-less Broccoli Cheddar Quiche   74
Savory Steamed Egg Custard   76
Shakshuka (Poached Eggs in Tomato Cumin Sauce)   77
Artichoke Leek Frittata   78
Tex-Mex Scrambled Eggs   79

Salads and Vegetable Sides
Roasted Brussel Sprouts with Lemon Zest   81
Mushroom Fricassee   82
Zucchini Chips   83
Sautéed Broccoli Rabe   84
Roasted Spaghetti Squash and Meatballs   85

Kale Chips   87
Caprese Salad   88
Cauliflower Fried Rice   89
Summer Beef and Veggie Medley   90
Sunset Veggie Medley   91
Grilled Zucchini   91

Chicken, Turkey
Mesquite Rubbled Turkey Legs   93
Curried Chicken Soup   94
Lemon Chicken with Sugar Snap Peas   95
Asian Chicken Skewers   96
Chicken and Purple   97
Rosemary Balsamic Chicken   98
Asian Pineapple Chicken Stir- Fry   99
Chinese Honey Chicken Stir-Fry with Cashews   99
Stewed Louisiana Chicken Drumstick   100
Low carb Chicken Tenders   101
Kale Caesar with Chicken and Crispy Artichokes   102
Grilled Chicken Paillard Salad   104
Asian Peanut Noodles with Chicken   105
Baked Italian Chicken Breast   105

Meats
Pan Seared Sirloin Steak with Thyme and garlic   108
Chinese 5 Spice Pork Tenderloin   108
Jazzed up Steak and Eggs   109
Chinese Stir- Fry Beef with Bell Peppers   110
Grilled Herb Lamb Chops   111
Low Carb Meatballs   112
Shepard's Pie with Cauliflower Mash   113
Pernil (Cuban Roasted Pork Shoulder)   114

Fish and Shellfish
Octopus Salad   116
Grilled Salmon Collar   117
Mediterranean Grilled Octopus   118
Sesame Ahi Tuna   119
Seared Scallops   120
Shrimp with Healthy Plant Mix   121
Shrimp taco in Chickpea Tortilla   122
Baked Salmon with Mustard Dill Sauce   123
Almond Parmesan Crusted Cod   123
Pan Seared Red Snapper with Lime Cilantro Sauce   124
Grilled Whole Trout   124
Steamed Fresh Tilapia with Scallions and Ginger   125

Baked Goods
Chickpea Tortillas   128
Cauliflower Pizza Crust   129
Almond Flour Cheddar Biscuits (Low Carb)   130
Oopsie Bread   132
Lemon Almond Pound Cake   133
Low Carb Chocolate Bundt Cake   134
Low Carb Bread   135
Zucchini Noodles with Creamy Avocado Pesto   136
Closing Sentiments   138

Meet Mimi Chan, RD, LD, CNSC, CDE:

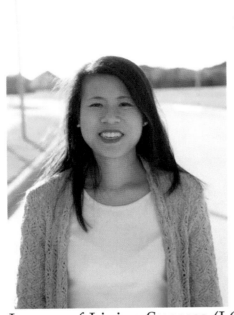

"My passion for food was always present even before my career path as a dietitian was on the horizon. I earned my Bachelor of Science degree from New York University. After graduation, I completed my training at New York Presbyterian Queens and remained part of their staff for the duration of my career. My reason for pursuing this career lies in this belief: the intimate relationship we have with what we put in our body should help us live a fruitful, healthy life, and not one that equates to daily medications, medical treatments and foreign procedures. Through my passion and respect for food and the belief in upholding quality of life, I have found a way to marry the two into a unique relationships through the creation of Layers of Living Success (LOLS). I believe that your mindset before a meal is more important than the next bite of food in your mouth. In this system, I strive to protect your traditions and your health through the use of food."

-Mimi Chan, RD, LD, CNSC, CDE
Find more about Mimi at Facebook.com/
mimichanfood
Tweet Mimi **@mimichanrd** on Twitter
Instagram: **@mimichanrd**
Website: NutritionComfort.com

Meet Dr. Cheng Ruan:

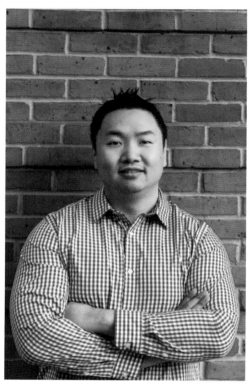

"I am a board certified Internal Medicine Physician who believes that the power of a conversation between a patient and his/her physician has far more impact than a quick prescription. I am a proud father of 2, a loving husband to a wife who is much smarter and better looking than I am, and a son of two physician parents who always reminded me to treat people and not to treat diseases. Coming from a large family of physicians who practice Traditional Chinese Medicine, I was always taught to use food to heal and exercise to nourish. Using food as medicine is not only a part of my life but it is also what I preach. I am the co-creator of the Layers of Living Success Type 2 Diabetes Reversal program (full edition included in this book)."

-Dr. Cheng Ruan, MD
Find more about Dr. Ruan at

Facebook : facebook.com/healthydoc/
Twitter: @theruanway
Pinterest : Theruanway
Instagram : dr.chengruan
Website : RuanMD.com
RuansHouse.com (for products and books Dr. Ruan Loves)
Subscribe to my Youtube Channel:
youtube.com/channel/UClBuvpXxUxt1jG4zHvFL1RQ

Introduction to
Layers of Living Success (LOLS)
The Story Behind the Creation
by: Dr. Cheng Ruan, MD

This **Diabetes Reversal Plan** started when I noticed something good happening to my patients. A few of my patients got their act together soon after the diagnosis of Type 2 diabetes, and they were able to get their average blood sugar down into the normal range in about 3-6 months. I was curious to see how this could be happening. At that time, it was a rarity to see people diligent enough to do something like this. I remember the first time I had a patient come into my office. When he came to my office, his hemoglobin A1c, which is the average blood sugar over 3 months, was 11.2 at that time. In about 3 months, he lost about 42lbs and his A1c dropped down to 5.2. The normal range of hemoglobin A1c is below 5.7 for non-diabetics, 5.7-6.4 for pre-diabetics, and 6.5 and above for diabetics. For this gentleman to drop his average blood sugar this far into a normal range was, quite frankly, unheard of for me. How was he able to do this when so many others had failed? How was he able to achieve what 99.9% of other people could not? To satisfy my curiosity, I had a deeper discussion with him and discovered there were certain principles that he adhered to, to be able to do this.

First, he kept track of everything that he ate. Second, he had a daily goal of what he wanted to eat and pre-planned to carry it out. Third, he had a high amount of food knowledge. This gentleman was an engineer, so he was already highly organized. This background gave him the advantage of making spreadsheets for his food intakes, tracking his weight, as well as his waist size. As daunting as all this seems to be for a lot of people, tracking his health allowed him to set daily goals and the ability to modify his daily goals as he went along.

I started to ask my other patients to do very similar things, not as in making spreadsheets but tracking. Most people have a hard time tracking their food, but I saw some had enough diligence to accomplish this. The more diligent they were able to track their food, the more success they had. This is not surprising by any measures since the road to success requires constant reassessment of our current position, whether it be in health, business, sports, or anything else that may matter to us.

Tracking alone is not going to be enough. There needs to be a system where we have to understand what each type of food does as it enters our body. Tracking plus knowledge of this system is the ultimate way to be successful. After these two patients, I diagnosed my father with Type 2 diabetes. Although his blood sugars were not that high, it was just on the other side of the diabetes range. He, too, was able to get his A1c down into the normal range and become essentially un-diabetic within 3 months. For an Asian man to give up rice is a big deal, but he did it because he had fundamental food knowledge. My father is blessed with the knowledge of being a physician. In fact, he's got one more doctorate than I do; he's an MD, Ph.D or PhD. Using his food knowledge, daily tracking and blood sugar tracking, he was able to get his blood sugar down to where he no longer needs any medication.

At this point, I feel that all my diabetic patients should have a fundamental understanding of food. I have changed the way I practice medicine since the day I diagnosed my father with Type 2 diabetes. I spend more time talking to my patients, trying to understand what their relationship with food is and how they are able to bring about their success.

It was the beginning of the Type 2 Diabetes Reversal program in this very book that you are reading. In 2015, I asked my friend, Mimi Chan, a Registered Dietitian, about how we can create our own system, one which is easy for people to understand, to obtain food knowledge and for them to put into practice the right away. During this period, we did have a lot of tug of war, lots of back and forth, about how we are going to do this. Ultimately, we decided to go with an approach that's unlike any other system. Instead of eating less or limiting portions of a diet plan, we had a reverse psychology method. We have a system where we have 6 different categories of food and the first three categories are virtually *unlimited*. In fact, not only is there not a maximum intake of those three categories, there are actually minimum intakes of those three categories. The categorization of food is based on the combination of the concept of the glycemic index, harmonized with other different models and theories of insulin resistance.

As we made our first version of the **Diabetes Reversal Program**, it was apparent that it was difficult for people to grasp this concept of eating a minimum amount of food rather than maximum amount of food. Most people understand diet as a limitation of different things. System that is limited.

The focus remains directed on having food availability of the categories that are NOT limited in our system. Instead of me telling you not to think of a pink elephant, I would tell you to think of a gray flamingo. If I were to tell you not to think of a pink elephant, you would definitely think of a pink elephant; but by diverting your attention to a gray flamingo, you would think of the gray flamingo and the pink elephant would never appear in your mind in the first place. This is the approach we want to put in place. Ultimately, diets are temporary by definition. Our system allows people to gain a fundamental knowledge of food and allows people to establish permanency in success through the way that they eat.

Thus we are very proud to present to you our Layers of Living Success: A Diabetes Reversal System that is detailed in this book. I hope you enjoy it as much as we enjoyed making it.

The Human Psyche –
First Step in Diabetes Reversal
by: Dr. Cheng Ruan, MD

This program was created with the focus of humans in mind. Humans, from the time we wake to the time we go to sleep, seek reward every second we are awake. Whenever we seek reward, we tend to take it from wherever we can get it. Throughout modern times, a reward became food. As food became readily available, we transitioned to seek food that was rich in sugar and processed sugar. When processed sugars became cheaply made and easily available worldwide, the epidemic of diabetes began.

Now, we humans are funny creatures; cognitively we understand what we need but we still feed into our instincts and desires. We understand there are things that are healthy and unhealthy for us. Yet more often, we continue to make choices that are deemed bad. Why is that? Why do we keep making these choices if we understand that whatever we're doing can be damaging to our body? Why do smokers continue to smoke, knowing that it is a major contributor of heart disease and strokes? Why do diabetics continue to eat sugary and high carb foods when they understand that it will raise their blood sugars, ultimately leading to organ damage and cardiovascular disease? Why is it that we behave in such ways that may be detrimental to our health? The short answer is that it's just something humans do. Humans seek reward and this reward system can be so strong that, cognitively, we may not be able to bypass it. The reward system is so strong it can become habitual behavior. Habits by definition are automatic, emotionless things that we do not think about when we act. Through certain formed habits, we feed into our body's deterioration. It's through these habits that we continue to suppress our lifelong goals because of this one defining attribute. We humans are addicted to instant reward and gratification.

Take this example - do you ever wonder why you go to a gym and the people you see there, day in and day out, are already fit? You think to yourself, "They don't need to be at the gym. They're already fit. They should be doing something else instead of spending hours at the gym". So, why is it that they continue to go to the gym? The reason is those people who are at the gym, day in and day out, use something different as a reward. They have a reward system in their brain that's focused on being fit. Now, I am not telling everyone reading this to be at a gym; it is just an example of why humans do certain things and explain how much of an influence our reward system has on us. No one is born without a reward system. A reward system is developed based on attaching things we do to a reward in order to reinforce how we can continue to help ourselves.

Here's another example of the reward system in action. You go to a restaurant and notice this scene. People, who appear to be fit and thin, order healthier options and the people, who appear to be less fit, order less healthy options. Cognitively, we understand that the people who are less fit need to have healthier options to get to where they want to be, but, once again, it's the reward system affecting their choices. The people who are less fit, naturally have a reward system based on habits that contribute to less healthy results for their body. The people who are already physically healthy and fit have a reward system of habits that promote their physique. We are all a result of how we built our reward system.

One last example is to look around the supermarket. You're grocery shopping and you notice other people's baskets or shopping carts. People who appear fit have healthier items in the shopping cart while those who appear less fit tend to pick out less nutritious options. Our habits and reward system are so intertwined; it even affects our shopping patterns.

In these few examples, we can see that habits and intentions do not seem to flow in the same direction every time. This is a very important concept to acknowledge if we want to alter our health's course. It's through understanding our psyche and our human behaviors that we can begin to move in the right direction.

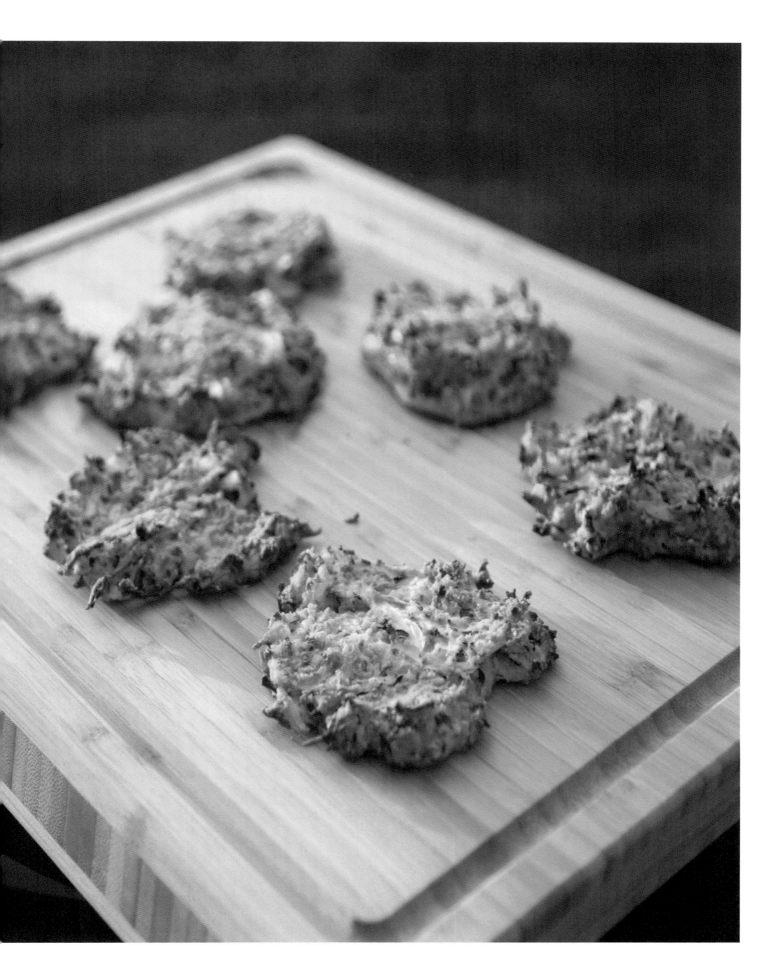

Why the Layers of Living Success (LOLS)?
By: Mimi Chan, RD, LD, CNSC, CDE

How many of these terms have you heard before? Carbohydrates, fiber, lean protein, glycemic index, microvascular risk, macrovascular risk, insulin resistance, saturated fats, monounsaturated fats, whole grains, vegetables, processed foods, carbohydrate counting, lancets, glucometers, beta-cells, adipose tissues, and I can go on. If you're a healthcare professional, these terms are used day in and day out when you're dealing with diabetes mellitus as a general category. If you're a person who has Type 2 diabetes, nine times out of ten, these terms will tend to bring on more stress and glazed looks. Why? Because these were foreign, science-based terms that were forced on you when you received your diagnosis. Right off the bat, you see diabetes and yourself as two separate beings because all these new terms are presented to you and you're expected to soak it up like new friends. Therein lies the problem: this is a completely new language, and not everyone is a linguist.

Diabetes can affect any person at any given time and does not choose you just because you have a science degree. Here lies the great disconnect. How do you bridge the science and unfamiliar cold facts into a realistic lifestyle for the average person to embrace? From a practical standpoint, I can tell you how great it is that vegetables will improve your blood sugar, provide fiber, nutrients and everything else foreign and intangible in those matter-of-fact statements. The great disconnect lies in how it fails to translate into a lifestyle a person can follow from each day forward.

You're thinking, "You must be mistaken! There are so many different systems out there to teach you how to live with diabetes!" Well, the answer is yes, there are plenty of systems geared towards helping you manage your health such as carbohydrate counting which is a method supported by the American Diabetes Association, point systems, specific diets such as Weight Watchers, DASH, Mediterranean, Atkins, and so on. This brings me to two questions I want to ask you. Why is the prevalence of diabetes still so high at an estimated 422 million people worldwide with this condition being the leading cause of death in the world? [1] More specifically, why do you still have Type 2 diabetes?

Now, if you are reading this book, I'm sure you're no stranger to the many different plans circulating around. If you did a search on how many different diets exist in the world today, nonspecific to diabetes, there are well over 600 different diets in circulation from your familiar carbohydrate counting to as catchy sounding as using numbers like 321 or 10 days or 21 days until your absolute dream comes true. You've likely tried them all and purchased their supplements, bought their products just to ensure you're eating the "right" types of foods, and were even told to live a different culture because the nutrition benefits are all there if you eat like they do! That probably sounds wonderful in the beginning and yes it will get you from point A to point B. However, what happens after point B and beyond? What happens once you shed the weight or get your HgbA1c down? Can this be a forever lifestyle just as strongly as your identification of yourself? Is this as natural of an integration as the idea of how you first learned food? That's the catch. It means nothing if we have the data and the methods but have a non-user friendly vehicle to deliver it. This is the impression I gathered after experiencing the frustrations from people living with Type 2 diabetes and after the review of the research available in the past few decades. There has to be a better way, and all of the reasons mentioned earlier were the driving force for the creation of the Layers of Living Success.

This lifestyle is created using the extraction of data and study results geared towards Type 2 diabetes and translating it to an intuitive eating pattern, placing food at the forefront versus the heavy science push that's been presented to you. The reason to rethink this approach is based on the premise that if the dietary guidelines were so easy to understand and the lifestyle was easy to follow, how is it that Type 2 diabetes, insulin resistance and obesity rates keep rising astronomically? Is the information too overwhelming to digest or is it that we, as healthcare professionals, are presenting two extremes of the information to the public? One extreme is being super narrow down to the micronutrient and highlighting only that nutrient for the public to focus on. The other extreme is conveying a message too broad, such as eat more real food and less processed foods, which leaves them directionless on how to translate this piece of advice into day-to-day life. Hence, this foundation is used to start on redefining how you look at food, starting with the theory of how you first learned about food from day one.

No matter what walk of life you came from, your first idea of food was given to you by someone who raised you, whether it be your parents, grandparents, family members, caretakers, etc. Your first experience with food was just the simple idea that you were hungry, and someone placed food in front of you. Next, you processed how it visually appealed to you, followed by how it tasted. Finally, you retained those memories of taste itself and your emotional attachments, whether it be of comfort, sadness, enjoyment, disgust or otherwise. As you accumulated more information about the food world all the while putting different types into your body, you build up compartments of stored information – your personal food dictionary.

Some people are better than others at connecting all the information points to one central idea. However, we cannot assume that everyone learns or operates in the same way. For example, when you see a piece of tuna– I'm almost certain your first thought will not be, "Oh, that's a lean protein, rich in omega-3 fatty acids, as well as rich in selenium, niacin, Vitamin B12 and phosphorus, but also a risk of high mercury content since it's a deep water fish, so I should limit it to six ounces per week." Yes, tuna has all those qualities, but even the most educated professional's first response to seeing tuna is simple – "Do I feel like eating this today or not, and why." The Layers of Living Success lifestyle is to bring the idea of food back to the basics of simple meal decisions – letting you decide what you want for each meal by re-categorizing foods into six different categories, teaching you how to build your food knowledge one meal at a time, as it highlights the reversal benefits of Type 2 diabetes in the background.

Another major barrier for people living with diabetes is learning about portions. Portion control and calorie restriction have shown great results in Type 2 diabetes. First, let us focus on calorie restriction. In 2012, Sarah Nowlin and her colleagues reviewed the existing literature to compare various diets and effects on inflammation in people with Type 2 diabetes. One of the results they found was that very low-calorie diets did help weight loss and helped decrease some inflammation, but the diet was not sustainable and supported the idea that rapid weight loss alone may not be beneficial for your long-term health.[2] In addition to this, the Look Ahead trial was published in 2013 comparing a very low-calorie diet to current diabetes education to see which one would help with weight loss to decrease cardiovascular disease (CVD) events in the diabetes population.

This was a large study that involved 5,145 overweight or obese individuals with Type 2 diabetes from 16 different centers across the United States over an average of almost ten years. What the researchers gathered is that the calorie restriction increased physical activity each week did assist with their weight loss, but it did not cut down the rates of cardiovascular (heart disease) events from happening. A limitation the researchers acknowledged was that they focused only on calories, and did not look at the food component itself.[3] A calorie is not just a calorie. As you see here, when you focus on the microscopic extreme, it does not translate to an overall effect. Life itself is not made up of one nutrient, or one day or one idea, so why should we expect anything different from everything else?

Next, you have portions of food, and different types of foods have different portion sizes. This in itself is a whole education experience. Carbohydrates, whether starch, fruit, dairy or sweets, all have different portion sizes that equal one serving of carbohydrate. Protein, whether it is lean or fatty have different portion sizes depending on the calorie range. Fat has its own and so on and so forth. No wonder people are frustrated with their meals! It's stressful and scary enough to receive the diagnosis, but next you have to solve math problems consciously with every single bite you take. This is where the portion sizes can be simplified to a more user-friendly method by using your hand as the measurement device.

Here's where you're going to get the inside scoop on one of the biggest secrets in the field. Daily calorie requirements are at best an estimation using various factors, such as age, height, weight, gender, activity, to come up with what you need to sustain in day to day activity. If you're able to get your hands on a metabolic cart, you may get a more accurate estimation, but that's again a snapshot in time. As you do different things at different times, your body adjusts to those changes. Will you ever know how much you need exactly down to the single digits of caloric requirements? Possibly, but as you saw before, a calorie is not just a calorie. As an observation in practice, I have noticed that your hand may be the best tool to individualize to your needs.

The Academy of Nutrition and Dietetics has long been teaching the public and dietitians to use your hand as an estimation tool. However, it always recommended you to look at a woman's hand for estimation sizes: one fist is approximately one cup, one palm size or a deck of cards is approximately three ounces and one thumb tip is approximately one teaspoon. Using this principle, the theory of using everyone's hand as an estimation tool came to light. Caloric requirements are different for everyone, and some need more than others. In efforts to provide people suffering from Type 2 diabetes with the most nutrients geared towards weight loss, decreasing insulin resistance, improving meal satisfaction and lowering complication risk factors, you will use your hand as your tool. My observation is that as gradual weight loss occurs, you may notice your hand changing sizes or, if you wear jewelry, your ring getting looser. This is the theory. At that given time, your body will gradually adjust to what you need to feel fulfilled while still maintaining this lifestyle as you progress day to day.

Now, just because it's easier to think about food and that measurement is no longer a problem doesn't mean that that's all there is to the Layers of Living Success. Compliance is a hot word amongst professionals all across the board. Lots of things are considered before a treatment plan is formed but what goes through every practitioner's mind each time is the word compliance. How compliant is someone going to be with diet, medication, lifestyle modification, a cessation plan, and so on? Or, on the flipside, how noncompliant someone is with the medical advice, such as any therapy and lifestyle changes implemented? Simply put– how likely is it that the person will do it? Well, that's where there was extra effort placed in the creation of the Layers of Living Success.

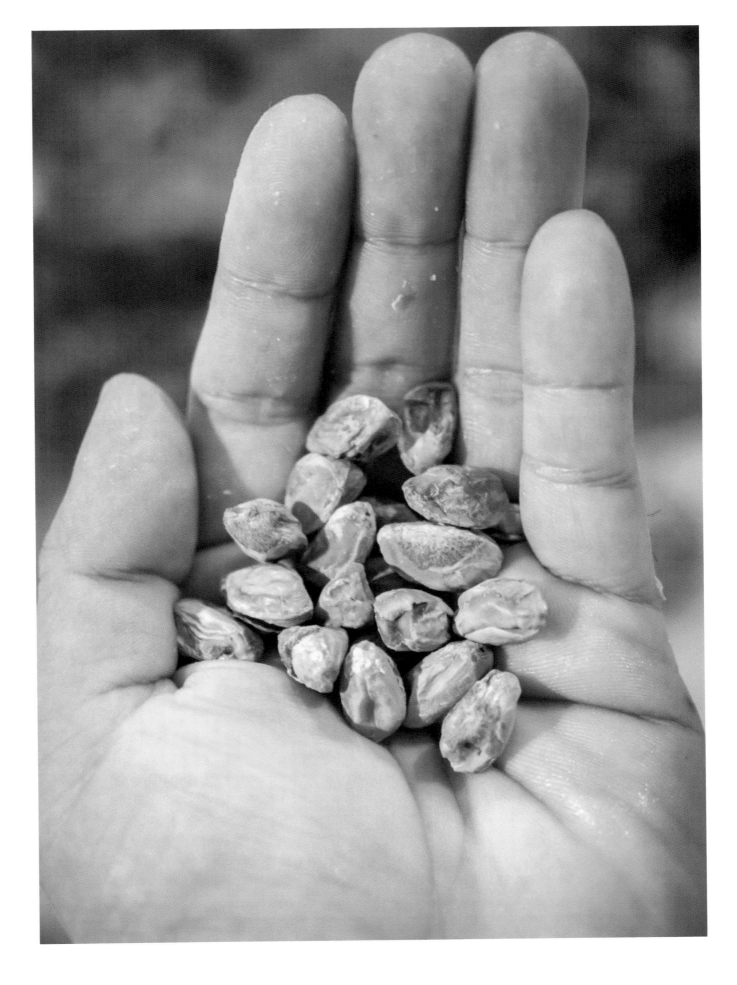

Creation of the
Layers of Living Success (LOLS)
By: Mimi Chan, RD, LD, CNSC, CDE

The Layers of Living Success is food re-categorized into six different categories or what we call layers. These six layers were created to build a foundation of food knowledge that helps you understand how it will help you decrease your insulin resistance. Therefore, over time, this will be the guiding factor in your Type 2 diabetes reversal. Insulin resistance is only one of many different factors considered when this system was built. There are several key items that are connected to Type 2 diabetes and success in this area needs to account for those items. They include **decreasing your insulin resistance, weight loss in people who are considered overweight (BMI greater than 25) or obese (BMI greater than 30), lowering cardiovascular disease (CVD) risks (due to this complication being a "primary cause of death in diabetes"), decreasing inflammation factors, and, decreasing complications related to Type 2 diabetes by lowering your blood sugar levels or hemoglobin A1c to less than 7% (53 mmol/mol).** [4]

Insulin is a hormone produced by your pancreas that normally helps take the sugar swimming around in your bloodstream into the tissue and organs to use as energy. The most common term is the "lock and key" model, where insulin is the key to open the doorway into the cells in your tissue and organs in order to bring the sugar molecules through. The easiest way for food to convert to sugar in your body is carbohydrates. There is one of two choices that happens in your muscles and tissues once the insulin has taken the sugar molecule in use the sugar as energy or store it as fat. In Type 2 diabetes, one of the defining characteristics is insulin resistance, or your body has become less sensitive to allowing insulin to take sugar into the body to use as energy. Lean tissue, such as muscle, is the most sensitive and fat is the least sensitive. Over a period of time, when your supply of food is more than what you use, it can deposit as fat, also known as adipose tissue. High levels of adipose tissue surrounding or intermixed into the lean tissue create a resistant environment. In Type 2 diabetes, it is not that you're not producing insulin, but in fact, you are producing a large amount of insulin to handle the continued intake of food you're placing into your body. The reason the sugar stays elevated is that what used to be sensitive is now resistant, and thereby your body has no choice but to let the levels build up and find other ways to get rid of your excess supply. The threshold of when your body can't handle the environment of elevated blood sugars is when you cross over to Type 2 diabetes.

Researchers over the past 46 years have studied various characteristics found in people who live with Type 2 diabetes in hopes of addressing all the items mentioned earlier. In the review of the most recent literature combined with the most recent clinical practice guidelines of the American Association of Clinical Endocrinologist (AACE) and American College of Endocrinology (ACE) for diabetes mellitus care, we pulled out pieces of the puzzle and stored little "nuggets" of findings to create this Type 2 diabetes reversal plan.[4]

In addressing insulin resistance, let us first look at how to take care of the fat content or adipose tissue. Dr. Gerald Reaven is an endocrinologist who is most widely known for his work on diabetes research. In his collaborative work with colleagues' in 2004, they found a clear distinction needed to be made between Type 2 diabetes, obesity, and insulin resistance.[5] While looking at the ever climbing overweight/obesity problem in the adult population, there was a large portion of people who were insulin resistant.[5] The distinction that Reaven et al. pointed out is not every single overweight/obese person is insulin resistant. Several tell-tale characteristics that were found in insulin resistance in overweight/obese people are glucose tolerance issues, high insulin levels, dyslipidemia (or poor lipid profiles such as triglycerides, LDL, etc.) and high C-reactive protein levels (an inflammation marker). With the combination of insulin resistance and increased fat tissue in overweight/obese people, there was a much larger risk of CVD development due to metabolic deviations.[5] Weight loss seemed to bring on the most effective benefits in addressing all the deviations related to insulin resistance and CVD risk.[5] In efforts to bring insulin sensitivity back to people living with Type 2 diabetes, weight loss is a goal that's placed into this reversal plan.

However, one calorie is not the same as another calorie. Weight loss alone did not address the decrease in CVD rates as seen in the Look Ahead Trial.[3] After close to ten years of observation in this study, the researchers found no significant reduction in CVD events from an intensive lifestyle change using calorie restriction and exercise versus standard diabetes education.[3] What is interesting to note is that the researchers did acknowledge that while they "used a specific lifestyle that focused on achieving weight loss through caloric restriction and increased physical activity, it is unclear whether an intervention focused on changes in dietary composition might have different outcomes.[3] This is another nugget of information to investigate. Weight loss in insulin resistance can help improve the parameters related to resistance, helping the body become more insulin sensitive, but the method of weight loss seems to need more attention. This is the start of how the six layers of food were created for the Layer of Living Success. The focus is aimed towards not looking at calorie counting and specific isolated nutrients, but an encompassing system to allow you to choose foods best suited for insulin resistance reduction, weight loss, lowering CVD risk, inflammation factors, and also decreasing diabetes-related complications by using food as your vehicle to push your hemoglobin A1c to less than 6.5% (48 mmol/mol).

Each layer of food is categorized based on the critical role it plays in Type 2 diabetes reversal and is essentially built to almost a tier system, for the highest on your priority down to the lowest. Layer 1 is coined the "unlimited layer". Vegetables and herbs have long been public knowledge to provide health benefits. These plant-based foods contain phytonutrients, antioxidants, and fiber of varying caliber. A 2010 analysis was conducted to look at what specific roles diet and lifestyle contributed to diabetes prevention from the existing research in those last ten years.[6] In the review of numerous studies in this analysis, the researchers came to a conclusion that antioxidants from vitamin C and E, various flavonoids and carotenoids all added to a relative decrease in diabetes risk.[6] Certain types of nutrients were found to be low in Type 2 diabetes such as chromium and magnesium, but all the studies came back inconclusive when researchers isolated it down results. In the OMEGA trial which evaluated omega 3 fatty acid supplementation in the management of acute lung disease, the researchers also assumed that since omega-3 fatty acids had anti-inflammatory properties, it would help in improving oxygenation as well as improve by helping with the inflammatory state.[7] However, the conclusion was that it did not produce their desired outcomes. This brings the focus back to vegetables, the food itself. Broccoli, asparagus, green beans, mushrooms are chromium-rich foods. Dark leafy greens are rich in magnesium. On top of the flavonoids and carotenoids packed into various varieties of vegetables and herbs, they are lower in caloric range than all other foods known. From a culinary standpoint, they can be very versatile and filling. From a supply standpoint, if you're consuming to the point you consider full or satiated, there's less incentive to keep on eating more.

In consideration of the foods to include in Layer 1, there was also attention paid to meal planning and cultural standpoint. The concern of any lifestyle is that it has to be relevant to the person living it. Diabetes does not discriminate nor does it have a preference on which state or country it affects. It has become a worldwide issue and with populations being more diverse, especially with immigration, why should we only target an American diet, a Swedish diet, a Korean diet, a Mediterranean diet, a labeled plan? This is the first plan that we know of that attempts to place an emphasis with the user in mind. From my observations, the most common complaints from different populations about following the American Diabetes Association guidelines are, "you don't have my food. I don't eat 'American' foods."

In efforts to be culturally sensitive and to help those to recognize better eating methods with their familiar foods, we recategorized the foods from their standpoint to improve compliance. You're more likely to eat the foods you're familiar with rather than explore the unknown based on consumption habits. Using this belief, it can guide the user to create healthy meals with their familiar ingredients while still giving them options to explore other foods familiar to different cultures. Not everyone is open to the cold turkey method nor the likelihood of telling someone it's okay to offend my culture by saying, oh you have the worst foods in your culture for your diabetes, eat my way! Try having someone listen to you if you were on the receiving end of that remark!

Humans are very visual creatures, and it seems that seeing options can bring more inspiration than imagination. General recommendations such as "have a vegetable at every meal" does not sound as appealing nor lend to the imagination in terms of how to put together a meal. This is the reason for including such a vast list of different foods into this layer. There is a selection based on the taste profile, nutrition component, fiber, caloric level and cultural standpoint. Some of the foods on this list may not be familiar to you, but that's perfectly fine. These foods may be familiar to someone from a different culture and help them find their familiar traditions in their goals for diabetes reversal. The herbs, sauces, and a variety of vegetables are meant to inspire your culinary curiosity to give your meal time routine a little more fun. Hence, these foods are placed in the forefront for your attention. Also, it is worth noting that different spices were not included in the plan since everyone's seasoning preference is unique. Any spice that is not salt based is a welcome part of this diabetes reversal plan.

Layer 2 is called the preferred protein layer and it is filled with lean protein options. Adequate protein consumption is important in diabetes management. [8] This layer pays attention to separate protein choices to four categories: meat/poultry/game, lacto-vegetarian, pesco-vegetarian and vegetarian/vegan options. Legumes (also known as pulses and beans), found in the vegetarian/vegan option, is a type of food that has been associated with improving glycemic control and lowering CVD risks. [6],[8],[9] For these reasons, many different types were listed to bring about meal-time inspiration. Other options were also included for their nutrition profile, such as being rich in chromium and magnesium, and versatility in meal creations. As previous studies have shown, isolation and strict nutrition profiles did not lend to good compliance nor improvement in Type 2 diabetes. The goal of Type 2 diabetes reversal is not to be a diet but a lifestyle permanent and enjoyable. This is a guiding principle in how the rest of the layers are addressed.

Layer 3 is called the favorite fats layer. This layer addresses the foods that are high in monounsaturated fats, polyunsaturated fats, such as omega-3 fatty acids, and other foods made from such fats to promote glycemic control, anti-inflammatory benefits, and is an integral part of weight loss.[2],[6],[10],[11], [12] Fat tends to slow down gastric emptying, which is part of the digestion process, so one of the best qualities of fat is that it can help you curb hunger by suppressing your appetite. The types of foods found in this layer can range from oils to nuts and seeds as well as sauces based on a majority of these food items. Since this is an integral part of the diabetes reversal plan, it is highlighted as the third layer. These first three layers are not optional and are critical in the reversal process, which is why minimums were created to ensure you do not overly restrict yourself. As seen in other diets and calorie restrictions, the effect is short-lived and does not translate to a lifelong process. This is created with permanency in mind. The last three layers are where special consideration needs to be paid. Since carbohydrate rich food converts to sugar or glucose molecules in the highest concentration compared to protein and fat, the rest of the plan is aimed at decreasing the load through a low carbohydrate intake. Many prior studies of low carbohydrate diets compared to moderate carbohydrate, high carbohydrate and the American Diabetes Association dietary recommendations came to the conclusion that low carbohydrate intake tended to improve Type 2 diabetes related factors.[8],[10], [13] Again, as seen before, low carbohydrate was not the whole story. The glycemic index had an effect on how beneficial it was to Type 2 diabetes. This is the next addition to the diabetes reversal plan.

Layer 4 is called the low glycemic index layer. The glycemic index is a ranking of how foods that have carbohydrates affect blood sugars. The lower the ranking, the lower the effect on blood sugar rising. This layer is made up of various foods and sauces that have a low glycemic index value. At the same time, some of the sauces in these sections have a higher sodium level than previous layers, but still pack good flavor for meal creation. This is one of the reasons why these sauces are placed at a lower layer instead. As noted in previous studies, monounsaturated fats and other related higher fat intake options from Layer 3 tend to produce favorable results towards Type 2 diabetes. However, this effect is frequently seen when combined with low glycemic index diets.[14] In addition to looking at monounsaturated fats and low glycemic index diets, various other studies found that low carbohydrate tended to have larger weight loss capacity when combined with high fiber intake.[6],[10] In 2014, a randomized control trial was published testing out how the glycemic index affected weight loss, inflammation, satiety, and other risk factors. [15] In this study, they found that a low glycemic index diet improved fasting insulin levels, decreased insulin resistance and improved beta cell function (beta cells are found in your pancreas and are responsible for storing and releasing insulin).[15] All these little nuggets of information went into formulating this plan, but there's more to this puzzle.

In 2013, the Canadian Diabetes Association's guidelines included the recommendation of replacing high glycemic index foods with low glycemic index foods during meal time to improve glycemic control.[16] In their literature review, there was decreased triglyceride levels, decreased CVD risk, decreased medication reliance, improved post-meal blood sugars and also decrease C-reactive protein levels associated with this consumption pattern.[15] Why isn't the glycemic index part of all diabetes education then? Well, although it is recommended, it is "based on the individual's interest and ability".[15] I believe if the vehicle to deliver the information is user-friendly, half the work has already been done for you. Since this system is important in diabetes management, it was included to show you how it can translate to your own meal time inspiration instead of a mouth full of scientific terms.

Layer 5 is called the preferred carbohydrate layer. These types of carbohydrates choices have a higher glycemic index. However, they are still called preferred due to the antioxidants, flavonoids, carotenoids and fiber content that can be found in these foods. For example, whole grains are part of this section. In various studies, high fiber intake and whole grains tended to improve CVD risk factors such as abnormal lipid levels and glycemic levels, giving it a role in Type 2 diabetes management. [10],[14] Since the ultimate goal is to reverse diabetes, these foods have a role, but it's smaller compared to the other layers importance.

Layer 6 is what I like to call sparing the spare tire layer. This layer includes all the refined grains, processed foods, simple sugars, saturated fats and sodium-laced sauces that have all been associated with negative effects on Type 2 diabetes, obesity rates, heart disease and other health conditions. However, they are still included in Type 2 diabetes reversal. How is that possible? Well, in review of the literature and from clinical practice, people don't fare well with restrictions or a restrictive mindset, as seen in the calorie restriction studies. Even the AACE/ACE guidelines to achieving glycemic targets in Type 2 diabetes made a note to say that "adherence to the diet was the single most important criterion of successful weight loss" and the "key.. is to personalize the recommendations on the basis of a patient's specific medical conditions, lifestyle and behaviors."[4] My principle of a healthy lifestyle is knowing how to balance and co-exist with the presence of these foods while understanding that they don't contribute to your ultimate goal. As you live a low carb lifestyle, it can help reduce "sweet cravings, emotional eating, and improve self-discipline towards food in itself."[11] Through this empowerment, you take control into your hands.

Two more key points to address are inflammation reduction and getting your hemoglobin A1c to less than 6.5%. Type 2 diabetes has been recently looked at as an inflammatory disease in which a poor lifestyle (described as high added sugar intake, processed grains and saturated fats adding to excessive weight gain) can have an influence on this condition.[2] Inflammation can be stimulated by various situations such as "environmental, behavioral, individual, psychosocial or diet-induced from high blood sugar environments or high triglycerides."[2] Chronic levels of inflammation can lead to disease complications such as CVD and nephropathy (kidney damage).[2] In an effort to minimize inflammation stimulation, the layers were created to decrease inflammation from a food standpoint and a stress reduction standpoint. The theory is that if something as natural as eating becomes a stressful situation and negative emotions are associated with this action, it serves no purpose to push anti-inflammatory properties onto you.

Lastly is to understand hemoglobin A1c reduction. Your hemoglobin A1c level is based on how saturated your red blood cells are with sugar molecules. If your blood sugars are elevated consistently, it will latch onto your red blood cells. Since each red blood cell's life span is about 90 days, this is used as a marker to check how saturated your blood is with sugar molecules over three months. Diabetes-related complications stem from uncontrolled blood sugars. Patients with a hemoglobin A1c level greater than 7% tend to have a higher risk of microvascular (such as kidney disease and blindness) and macrovascular (CVD and stroke) complications. The AACE/ACE guidelines recommend an A1c level less than 6.5%, but only if it can be achieved safely. The basis of this recommendation is in a large part due to two major trials, the ACCORD and ADVANCE trials, aiming to reduce hemoglobin A1c using intensive medical regimens to bring down blood sugars in efforts to decrease complication risks.[17],[18] In these major studies, mortality increased when they attempted to treat the patients intensively and largely in part related to hypoglycemia.[4],[17][18] However, it is worth noting that neither of the studies focused on diet or lifestyle modification. Therefore, the approach of putting food first towards diabetes reversal became the plan. This does not mean you should not pay attention to your blood sugars nor should you be unaware of your medication regimen. This should still be on your radar so there can be effective communication between you and your doctor in your diabetes reversal goal.

Another unique characteristic of this plan is the built-in sliding scale eating pattern. Depending on what your blood sugars are that morning, you can utilize different portions or different partitions of each of the categories of food to improve those numbers. For those who have poorly controlled diabetes, check your blood sugar before each meal to glimpse how you're doing and how to create your next meal. This method will likely impact the next morning's blood sugar which hopefully will become lower by the way you eat the day before. The lower your blood sugar becomes, the more options you're allowed to choose. It becomes a reward system that's designed for success. As you are rewarded by lower blood sugars from your actions, you get to build in more "cheat" meals if the blood sugars remain low. However, if the blood sugars become higher the next morning or by the next meal, some of the layers are not available for that meal. Surprisingly, what we've noticed is that people do not opt for the "cheat" meals anymore because their reward becomes the lowered blood sugar results instead of being food. Therefore, since they don't want their blood sugars to go up again, they naturally avoid cheat meals.

Type 2 diabetes is a reversible condition, and you have the tools in you to accomplish this. This plan was created to address the frustrations seen in current practice, but mostly inspired by you, the person with Type 2 diabetes. You are a person first, who is not defined by diabetes, in which you have likes and dislikes, traditions and personalities like every other person. We distilled the science to bring you a more practical approach to healthy living through our approach to diabetes reversal. We hope this brings out the best version of you along this journey.

References

[1] 10 facts about diabetes. (2016, April). Retrieved from http://www.who.int/features/factfiles/diabetes/en/

[2] Nowlin, S. Y., Hammer, M. J., & Melkus, G. D. (2012). Diet, Inflammation, and Glycemic Control in Type 2 Diabetes: An Integrative Review of the Literature. *Journal of Nutrition and Metabolism, 2012*, 1-21. doi:10.1155/2012/542698

[3] Cardiovascular Effects of Intensive Lifestyle Intervention in Type 2 Diabetes. (2013). *New England Journal of Medicine N Engl J Med, 369*(2), 145-154. doi: 10.1056/nejmoa1212914

[4] Handelsman, Y., Bloomgarden, Z. T., Grunberger, G., Umpierrez, G., Zimmerman, R. S., Bailey, T. S., . . . Zangeneh, F. (2015). American Association Of Clinical Endocrinologists And American College Of Endocrinology – Clinical Practice Guidelines For Developing A Diabetes Mellitus Comprehensive Care Plan – 2015. *Endocrine Practice, 21*(Supplement 1), 1-87. doi:10.4158/ep15672.glsuppl

[5] Reaven, G. (2004). Obesity, Insulin Resistance, and Cardiovascular Disease. *Recent Progress in Hormone Research, 59*(1), 207-223. doi:10.1210/rp.59.1.207

[6] Psaltopoulou, T., Ilias, I., & Alevizaki, M. (2010). The Role of Diet and Lifestyle in Primary, Secondary, and Tertiary Diabetes Prevention: A Review of Meta-Analyses. *The Review of Diabetic Studies Rev Diabet Stud, 7*(1), 26-35. doi:10.1900/rds.2010.7.26

[7] Rice, T. W., MD, MSc, Wheeler, A. P., MD, Thompson, B. T., MD, DeBoisblanc, B. P., MD, Steingrub, J., MD, & Rock, P., MD, MBA. (2011). Enteral Omega-3 Fatty Acid, γ-Linolenic Acid, and Antioxidant Supplementation in Acute Lung Injury. *Jama, 306*(14), 1574-1581. doi:10.1001/jama.2011.1435

[8] Woo, M., Park, S., Woo, J., & Choue, R. (2010, July 23). A Comparative Study of Diet in Good and Poor Glycemic Control Groups in Elderly Patients with Type 2 Diabetes Mellitus. Retrieved from https://www.researchgate.net/publication/47791975_A_Comparative_Study_of_Diet_in_Good_and_Poor_Glycemic_Control_Groups_in_Elderly_Patients_with_Type_2_Diabetes_Mellitus

[9] Jenkins, D. J., Kendall, C. W., Vuksan, V., Faulkner, D., Augustin, L. S., Mitchell, S., . . . Leiter, L. A. (2014). Effect of Lowering the Glycemic Load With Canola Oil on Glycemic Control and Cardiovascular Risk Factors: A Randomized Controlled Trial. *Diabetes Care Dia Care, 37*(7), 1806-1814. doi:10.2337/dc13-2990

[10] Kodama, S., Saito, K., Tanaka, S., Maki, M., Yachi, Y., Sato, M., . . . Sone, H. (2009). Influence of Fat and Carbohydrate Proportions on the Metabolic Profile in Patients With Type 2 Diabetes: A Meta-Analysis. *Diabetes Care, 32*(5), 959-965. doi:10.2337/dc08-1716

References (Continued)

[11] Saslow, L. R., Kim, S., Daubenmier, J. J., Moskowitz, J. T., Phinney, S. D., Goldman, V., . . . Hecht, F. M. (2014). A Randomized Pilot Trial of a Moderate Carbohydrate Diet Compared to a Very Low Carbohydrate Diet in Overweight or Obese Individuals with Type 2 Diabetes Mellitus or Prediabetes. *PLoS ONE, 9*(4). doi: 10.1371/journal.pone.0091027

[12] Jenkins, D. J., Kendall, C. W., Vuksan, V., Faulkner, D., Augustin, L. S., Mitchell, S., . . . Leiter, L. A. (2014). Effect of Lowering the Glycemic Load With Canola Oil on Glycemic Control and Cardiovascular Risk Factors: A Randomized Controlled Trial. *Diabetes Care Dia Care, 37*(7), 1806-1814. doi:10.2337/dc13-2990

[13] Davis, N. J., Tomuta, N., Schechter, C., Isasi, C. R., Segal-Isaacson, C. J., Stein, D., . . . Wylie-Rosett, J. (2009). Comparative Study of the Effects of a 1-Year Dietary Intervention of a Low-Carbohydrate Diet Versus a Low-Fat Diet on Weight and Glycemic Control in Type 2 Diabetes. *Diabetes Care, 32*(7), 1147-1152. doi:10.2337/dc08-2108

[14] De Natale, C., MD, Ph.D., Annuzzi, G., MD, Bozzetto, L., MD, Mazzarella, R., MD, Costabile, G., Ph.D., Ciano, O., RD, . . . Rivellese, A. A., MD. (2009, September 9).Diabetes Care. Retrieved from http://care.diabetesjournals.org/lookup/doi/10.2337/dc09-0266

[15] Juanola-Falgarona, M., Salas-Salvadó, J., Ibarrola-Jurado, N., Rabassa-Soler, A., Díaz-López, A., Guasch-Ferré, M., . . . Bulló, M. (2014, April 30). The American Journal of Clinical Nutrition. Retrieved from http://ajcn.nutrition.org/content/100/15/27.full

[16] Dworatzek, P. D., Arcudi, K., Gougeon, R., Husein, N., Sievenpiper, J. L., & Williams, S. L. (2013). Nutrition Therapy. *Canadian Journal of Diabetes, 37*. doi: 10.1016/j.jcjd.2013.01.019

[17] Patel, A., MD, PhD, MacMahon, S., DSc, PhD, Chalmers, J., MD, PhD, Neal, B., MD, PhD, Billot, L., MSc, Woodward, M., PhD, . . . Travert, F., MD. (2008, June 12). Intensive Blood Glucose Control and Vascular Outcomes in Patients with Type 2 Diabetes — NEJM. Retrieved from http://www.nejm.org/doi/full/10.1056/NEJMoa0802987

[18] Dluhy, R. G., MD, & McMahon, G. T., MD, MMSc. (2008, June 12). Intensive Glycemic Control in the ACCORD and ADVANCE Trials — NEJM. Retrieved from http://www.nejm.org/doi/full/10.1056/NEJMe0804182

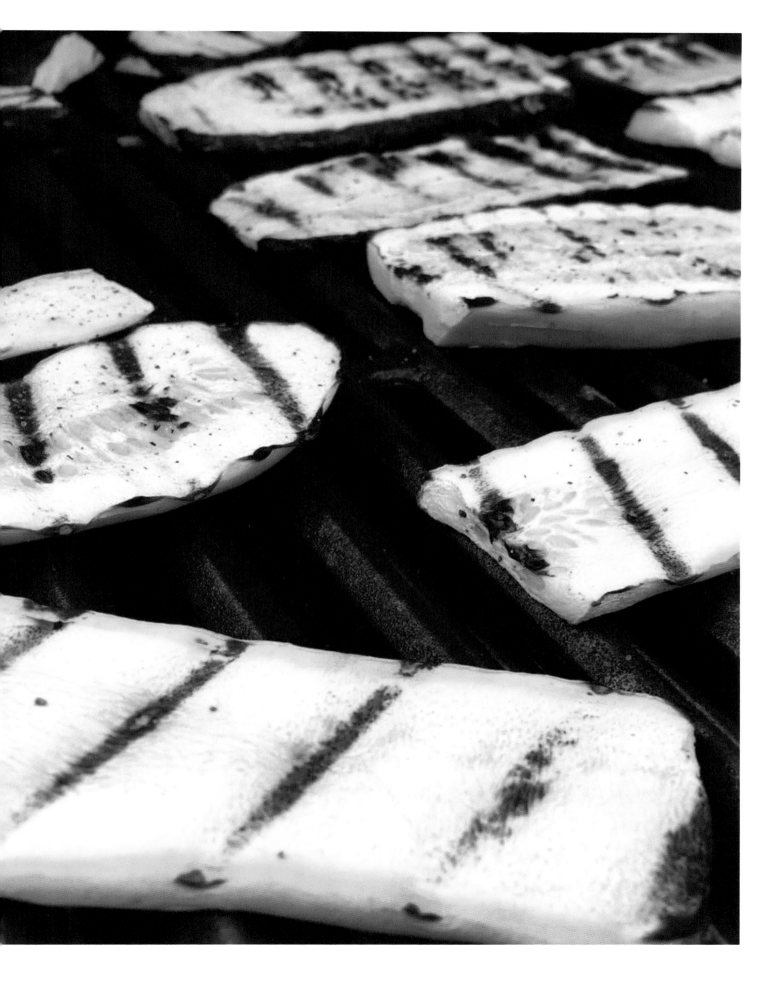

LAYERS OF LIVING SUCCESS
(LOLS)

A DIABETES REVERSAL PLAN

Dust Off Diabetes

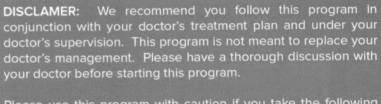

Please use this program with caution if you take the following medications due to risk of hypoglycemia (low blood sugar):

Sulfonylureas include Glyburide (Brand Names: Diabeta ®, Micronase ®, Glynase Prestab ®), Glipizide (Brand Names: Glucotrol ®, Glucotrol XL ®), Glimepiride (Brand Name: Amaryl ®), Chlorpropamide (Brand Name: Diabinese ®), Tolbutamide (Brand Name: Orinase ®), and Tolazamide (Brand Name: Tolinase ®).

Short Acting Insulins include Regular Humulin or Novolin and Velsosulin.

Rapid Acting Insulins include Lispro (Humalog), Aspart (Novolog) and Glulisine (Apidra).

This program is not meant for people who have the following: End stage kidney disease (ESRD), severe vision loss, coronary artery disease, cardiovascular disease, vascular diseases or hypoglycemia unawareness (tendency to not know when you have low blood sugar).

Dear Person with Type 2 Diabetes:

Are your blood sugars running higher and higher? Are you in need of more and more medications to get your sugars under control? Are you tired of living through this vicious cycle? Studies have shown that long periods of high blood sugars increase the chances of heart disease, high blood pressure, high triglycerides and high cholesterol. Over the last 10 years, many research studies have found that the approach we had towards diabetes management and weight loss needed to be looked at again. We have a solution that you have been looking for and it's been backed by research. It will likely make you feel better and you may have more energy!

Ask yourself. Do you want your health to be back on track? Do you want to feel better and stop piling on the pills? Then use the Layers of Living Success (LOLS) to help you reach your blood sugar goals. I will show you how you can do this in a few simple ways, starting with how you look at your foods. Your journey starts... now.

Sincerely,

Mimi Chan, RD, CDN, LD, CNSC, CDE
Chief Executive Officer
Dust Off Diabetes, LLC

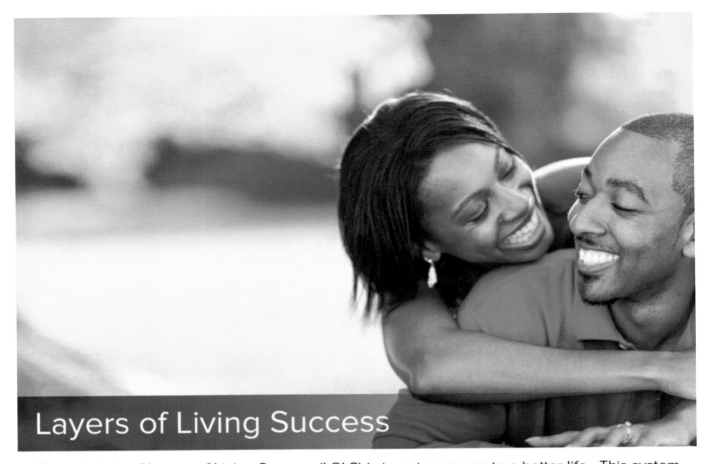

Layers of Living Success

The principle of Layers of Living Success (LOLS) is to eat your way to a better life. This system is meant to optimize your nutrition and spare you from breaking the sugar bank. The beauty of it: you get to eat for your blood sugar, choose smartly based on your goals and still be able to enjoy your meals. LOLS is a way of eating created to make eating well for our bodies as simple as possible. It highlights that nutrition should be your top priority.

Food has long been split into different categories like starches, fruits, vegetables, meats, and so on, but that doesn't always help meal planning. For example, an apple is great, but how much should you eat? LOLS helps you take out that guess work of having to measure and weigh your food. Let's face it. It's great to use measuring cups and food scales to weigh out exact portions, but that takes time. If you're already doing that, great; but for lots of people – it's an added burden. Eating well should never be a burden.

This is for you if you're:
• tired of measuring your food
• tired of trying to figure out what you should have
• tired of being tired

Welcome to Something Great!

Thank you for putting yourself and your health first! Many before you have been successful using this very plan to not only fully reverse Type 2 Diabetes and Prediabetes, but also to lose fat, decrease their bad cholesterol, and decrease triglycerides. Many have even eradicated their need to inject insulin! I am truly excited for you to commit to this plan!

How to Use the Layers of Living Success Plan

Understand that these "Layers" are like layers of foundation to a perfectly structured house. Layers 1 through 3 contain foods that are the foundation of what we are supposed to eat to help us reverse insulin resistance, and therefore helping to reverse Type 2 Diabetes and Prediabetes. Therefore, the foods in layers 1, 2, and 3 are unlimited. In fact, there are MINIMUMS we would like you to eat. The minimum quantities are at the top of the respective pages for each layer. The reasoning behind this is that as humans, we cannot survive on the concept of restriction lifelong. We seek reward from the moment we wake up to the moment we fall asleep. Since the first 3 layers are unlimited, always go to the foods in those categories if you're hungry or need snacking. This way, there is no guess work since there are no limits to those layers! Layers 4, 5, and 6 are LIMITED; the limited quantities are described in the top colored sections in the respective sections.

Layer 1 is a list of non-starchy vegetables which provide a huge boost of antioxidants (depending on what you eat), while providing big fillers with fiber and phytonutrients our bodies.

Layer 2 is a list of the protein sources divided into meats, seafood, and vegan sources of proteins like beans (this is my favorite layer).

Layer 3 is a list of fats! Remember, this is also limitless!

Layers 4 and 5 have a mixture of different categories of foods that are relatively limited. However, these two layers can be used if your blood sugars are in a specific range (described at the top of each page).

Layer 6 is the no-no zone! This layer is to be completely avoided for those on insulin and for those who have blood sugars above 200 (with or without insulin)!

The page with the pie charts represent a 9 inch plate of food, based on blood sugar range for that day. It is a suggestion of portion sizes when you look down on your plate. But remember, Layers 1, 2, and 3 are unlimited so feel free to pack them on! If you are instructed by your doctor to check your blood sugars once daily, then use your fasting blood sugar as references for the portion sizes. If you are checking multiple times a day as instructed by your doctor, use the blood sugar results before each meal as a reference point for portion sizes.

If you are on insulin, you may have a high change of having hypoglycemia (low blood sugar) so please work with your doctor on lowering your dose if this occurs!

If you are on sulfonureas such as glipizide, glimepride, glyburide, or on any combination drugs with these medications, note that you may also get episodes of hypoglycemia (low blood sugar) which can be life threatening. Please work with your physician to carefully adjust or even eliminate these medicines when using this eating plan!

"What if I have prediabetes and do not check my blood sugar?"

The way to use this plan without checking blood sugar is to adhere to the portion sizes at the top of each page. For layers 1-3, you would use the minimum portion sizes featured at the colored sections at the top of the plan. For layers 4 and 5, it would be limited to the portion sizes at the top of page (half a fist size three times a day for layer 4, and two times a day for layer 5). If your hemoglobin A1C does not change or even increase after 3 months, then go for stricter control by cutting out layers 5 and/or 6 altogether. Every body is different and it does take some time to learn how your body reacts to this plan.

Thank you!

Cheng Ruan, MD
Mimi Chan, RD, LD, CNSC, CDE

Visit DustOffDiabetes.com for more recipes and guidance!
Visit RuanMD.com for more health education and information!
Visit MimiChanFood.com for more tips from Mimi!

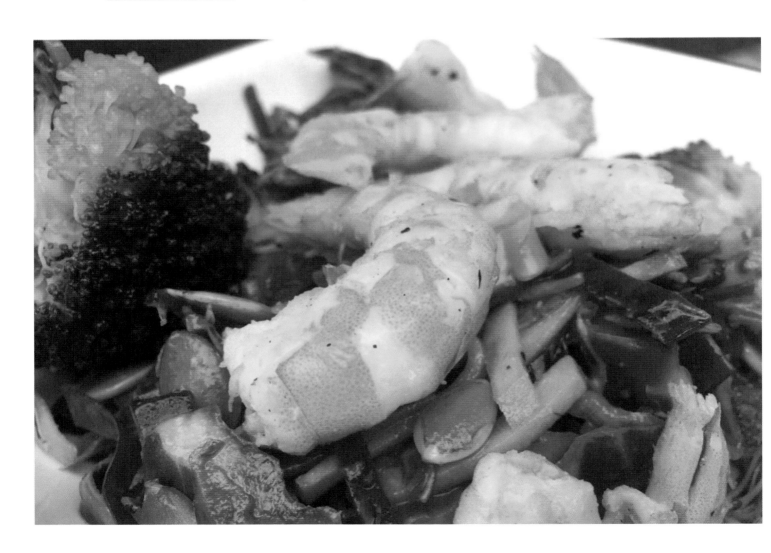

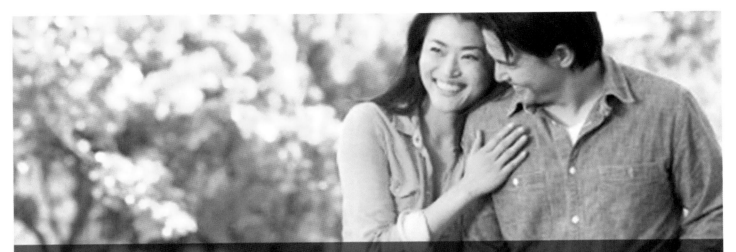

What is the Layers of Living Success?

LOLS has six layers, each with a variety of foods to choose from. Ranging from the top of your priority to the least of your concerns, there is something for everyone. Maintaining balance is our biggest enemy. These layers give you the balance you want without compromising your taste buds. Each layer teaches you what is preferred and how to eat for success. The layers are color coded to show you how it would look like on a plate, helping to take out a lot of the guess work.

Here are a few things you should know before getting started:

1. Always start with a 9-inch plate. This is the only measurement you need to take.

2. Look at your hand. Use your hand, not anyone else's. Remember this tip: **fist, palm, thumb.**

3. At every meal, you NEED TO EAT at least, NOT optional
    a. 1 fist size of Layer 1 (NEVER IGNORE, always have to have 1 fist but can be more)
    b. 1 palm size of Layer 2 (NEVER IGNORE, at least 1 palm but can be more)
    c. 1 thumb size of Layer 3 (NEVER IGNORE, at least 1 thumb but can be more)
    d. ½ fist size of Layer 4

4. Your meal should make sense to you
    a. Foods should appeal to your taste buds
    b. Foods should not look restrictive

5. Unsweetened beverages at every meal

The whole point of eating well is to eat for your blood sugars. Here are some tips on what your plates should look like based on your blood sugars before the meals.

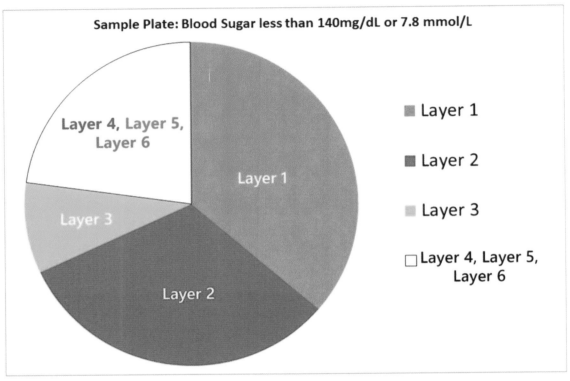

Sample Plate: Blood Sugar less than 140mg/dL or 7.8 mmol/L

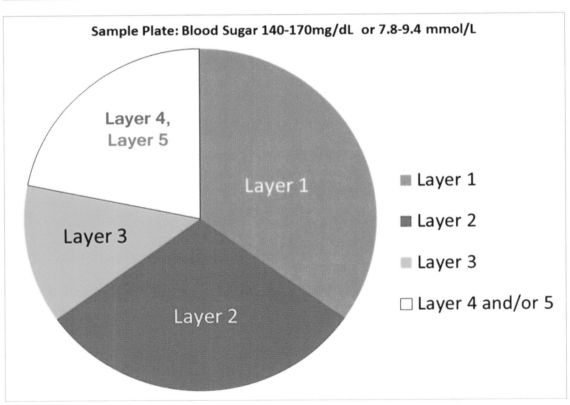

Sample Plate: Blood Sugar 140-170mg/dL or 7.8-9.4 mmol/L

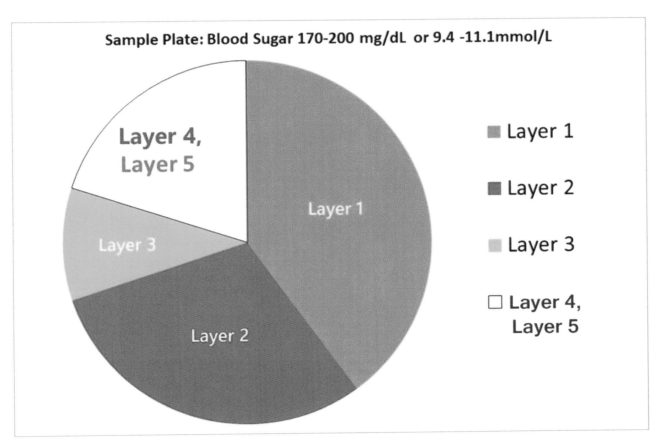

Sample Plate: Blood Sugar 170-200 mg/dL or 9.4 -11.1mmol/L

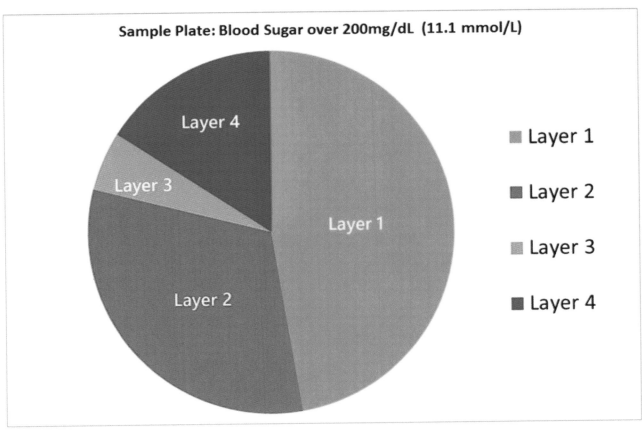

Sample Plate: Blood Sugar over 200mg/dL (11.1 mmol/L)

Layer 1: There's no daily limit. These are the foods that are usually neglected but have very high nutrition ratings. They are filling, tasty, attractive and the combinations are practically endless. The best part is you can eat all you want of these foods. This layer has something for everyone. You can find familiar foods or ideas for unfamiliar foods to introduce new tastes and textures to your world. There is even a special section for herbs and sauces that will flavor and brighten your meals. Also, it doesn't hurt that they are rich in antioxidants which helps protect the body.

If you have the chance to eat organic, give it a try. Your taste buds may surprise you.

Layer 1: No Daily Limit (High Value, Low on Health Cost)
NOT OPTIONAL - AT LEAST one fist size each meal (EXCEPT Sauces could be 3 thumb sizes and more)

Farm to Table

Alfalfa sprouts
Asparagus
Amaranth (aka Chinese Spinach)
Artichoke and artichoke hearts
Baby corn
Bamboo shoots
Beans
• Green Beans
• Italian Green Beans
• Wax Beans
Bean sprouts
Beets
Beetroot
Borcht
Braken Fern Stems (aka Fernbrake)
Broccoli
Brussel sprouts
Cabbage (all types including:)
Carrots (all colors)
Cauliflower (all colors)
Celery
Celeriac (aka celery root, knob celery or turnip-rooted celery)

Celeriac (aka celery root, knob celery or turnip-rooted celery)
Chives
Chayote
Cucumber (all types)
Eggplants
Escarole
Fiddleheads
Greens (many types)
Green Onions/Scallions
Gourds (many types)
Hearts of Palm
Jicama
Kohlrabi
Leeks
Lemon (all types)
Lettuce (all types)
Limes (all types)
Mung Bean Sprouts
Mushrooms (all types, fresh)
Nopal (AKA Nopale, prickly pear cactus pad/leaf)
Okra
Onions (all types)

Pea pods/Snow peas
Peppers (all types)
Purslane
Radish (all types)
Rapini (aka broccoli rabe)
Rutabaga
Rhubarb
Seaweed
Soybean sprouts
Spinach
Squash (many types)
Sugar Snap Peas
Swiss Chard
Tomatillo
Tomato (all types)
Turnips
Watercress
Water chestnuts
Yard long beans

Herbs

Basil (all types)
Bay Leaves
Blue Fenugreek
Curry Leaves
Cilantro
Caper
Chives
Chervil
Clary Sage
Dill
Elderflower
Epazote
Fennel
Fingerroot (Cambodian Ginger)
Garlic
Garlic Chives

Ginger
Horseradish
Jasmine Flowers
Juniper Berries
Kaffir Lime Leaves
Lavender
Lemon Balm
Lemon Verbena
Lemongrass
Marjarom
Mint
Oregano (Sweet, Cuban)
Pandan
Parsley
Peppermint
Rosemary

Sage
Shallots
Sorrel
Spearmint
Tarragon
Thyme (Regular, Lemon)
Wasabi

Sauces

Chili Garlic Sauce
Datil Pepper Sauce
Gremolata
Migonette
Mustard (NOT Honey Mustard)
Pico de Gallo
Salsa
Sofrito
Tabasco
Vinagrette
Worchestershire Sauce

Layer 2: Preferred Proteins. These foods are needed for daily function because they have important jobs in your body. They are known as the body's building blocks. They help build and repair our tissues. These proteins maximize your body's potential. They are also great for curbing hunger – they are filling and also have a low risk for spiking your blood sugars. The best way to prepare this layer is to have it steamed, grilled, baked, broiled, or even slow cooked. If you have the chance to eat organic, cage-free or both, try it.

Layer 2 (Preferred Protein)
NOTE: NOT OPTIONAL- AT LEAST your palm size (don't include fingers) for each meal

Meat/Poultry/Game

Buffalo
Chicken (skinless)
Cornish hen (skinless)
Domestic duck (drained of fat)
Domestic Goose (drained of fat)
Dove
Egg (whole, whites or substitutes)
Goat
Lamb (chop, leg, roast)
Lean beef cuts (might need trimming)
- ground round
- Roast (chuck, rib, rump),
- Round
- Sirloin
- Steak (cubed, flank)
- Tenderloin

Ostrich
Pheasant
Pork – rib or loin chop, roast, ham, tenderloin
Rabbit
Snake
Turkey (skinless)
Veal (loin, chop, roast)
Venison
Wild duck
Wild Goose
Deli Meats

Lacto-vegetarian

Cottage cheese

Pesco Vegetarian

Bass
Catfish
Clams
Cod
Crab
Croaker
Eel
Flounder
Gator
Geoduck
Haddock
Halibut
Herring
Lobster
Mahi-Mahi

Orange roughy
Oysters
Porgy
Roe
Salmon
Sardines
Scallops
Sea Urchin
Shrimp
Swai (Basa)
Swordfish
Tilapia
Trout
Tuna

Vegetarian/Vegan

Beans
- Black beans
- Cranberry beans
- Garbanzo
- Kidney beans
- Lima beans
- Navy beans
- Pinto beans
- Soy beans
- White beans
- Cannellini/Northern beans

Chickpea
Edamame
Lentils (brown, green, yellow)
Mock chicken/duck/pork/beef
Mung Beans
Nutritional Yeast
Peas (black-eyed, split, English, pigeon)
Red beans (AKA Adzuki Beans)
Soy based or pea-based products (burgers, "crumbles")
Spirulina
Tempeh
Tofu
Wheatgerm

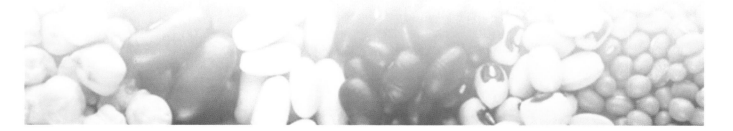

Layer 3: Favorite Fats. If these aren't your favorites yet, there's still time for you to get close to these gems. These foods help provide your body with the useful type of fats to maintain daily protection. It's great for your eyes, brain, and supports body functions like making hormones.

You can do many different things with these foods: cook them, spread them, eat them as is, or even use them as a mixer. They can add flavor and texture to any dish.

Layer 3: Favorite Fats
NOT OPTIONAL - AT LEAST one thumb size per meal

Fruits

Avocado
Durian
Olives
- Black
- Green
- Kalamata

Nuts

Almonds
Brazil
Cashews
Fiberts (Hazelnuts)
Macadamia
Peanuts
Pecans
Pistachios
Pignolia (Pine Nuts)
Walnuts (English)

Dairy

All non-processed cheese
Cream Cheese
Heavy Cream

Nut Butters/Spreads

Almond Butter
Cashew Butter
Peanut Butter
Grass Fed Butter
Mayonnaise

Oils

Corn Oil
Canola Oil
Cottonseed Oil
Flaxseed Oil
Grapeseed Oil
Olive Oil
Peanut Oil
Safflower Oil
Soybean Oil
Sunflower Oil
VIRGIN Coconut Oil

Fatty Meats

Bacon
Pork belly
Sausages
Fatty ground meats
Prosciutto
Jerky

Seeds

Chia seeds
Hempseed
Flaxseed
Pumpkin
Sunflower
Sesame seeds

Sauce

Beanaise Sauce
Chimichurri
Hollandaise Sauce
Mujdei (Garlic Sauce)
Persillade (Parsley Sauce)
Salsa Verde
Sauce Andolouse
Sauce Vierge

ONLY USE THIS IF YOUR BLOOD SUGAR FOR TODAY IS UNDER 200

Layer 4: Low Glycemic Index Foods. The key to your success in diabetes is to keep your blood sugars from spiking out of control. This layer introduces you to foods that are still carbohydrates (or carbs) but generally have a lower sugar spike risk than other carbs. These are the carbs to consider first when you're planning your meals.

This layer has many different types of foods and so it will be up to you to see what fits your taste buds. There are dairy choices, fruits, grains and even a low glycemic sweetener. There is also a special section for sauces you can choose to enhance your meals.

Layer 4 (Low Glycemic Index)
NOTE: ½ fist size each meal, EXCEPT if it's a sauce (then it's 1 thumb)
– MAXIMUM 3 times/day

Dairy

Greek Yogurt
Milk (Cow's, Whole)
Yogurt

Fruits

Acai Berry
Apple
Apricot
Banana
Berries (all types)
Grapefruit
Goii Berry
Longan Fruit
Nectarines
Orange
Peaches
Pear
Plums
Sour Cherries

Beverages

Soy milk (plain, unsweetened)
Almond milk (plain, unsweetened)

Grains

Barley (all types)
Brown Rice
Quinoa

Flour and flour-based foods

Coconut flour
Ezeikel bread
Mungbean noodles
Rice noodles
Rye
Soba Noodles
Porridge
  • Black rice
  • Rice bran

Vegetables

Acorns
Corn
Green Banana
Hominy
Hummus
Lotus Root
Burdock Root

Sweetner

Honey

Sauces

Fish sauce
Harissa
Hoisin sauce
Honey Mustard
Mala sauce
Oyster sauce
Pesto sauce
Plum sauce
Ponzu
Romesco
Sauce Gribiche (egg based)
Shito sauce
Soy sauce
Sriracha hot sauce
Tomato Paste
Tzatziki

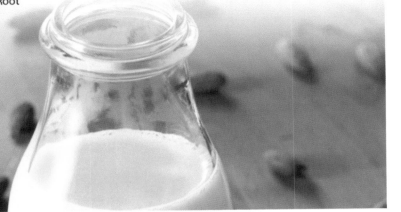

ONLY USE THIS IF YOUR BLOOD SUGAR FOR TODAY IS UNDER 200

Layer 5: Preferred Carbohydrates. This layer contains carbs that have a higher chance of spiking your sugar, but have preferred status because they still have a lot of nutritious value. These foods are packed with fiber and can feed your body the nutrients it craves. The catch is that overeating this level will curb your efforts to reverse diabetes.

This layer is similar to Layer 4. It has different choices like fruits, grains, vegetables and even certain type of sauces.

Layer 5 (Preferred Carbohydrates)
NOTE: ½ fist size, MAXIMUM 2 times/day
EXCEPT for Sauces (then it's 2 thumbs)

Fruit

Cantelope
Grapes
Guava
Honeydew
Jackfruit
Kiwi
Lychee
Mango
Papaya
Pineapple
Prickly pear
Watermelon

Sauce

Tomato Sauce
Marinara Sauce

Grains

Amaranth
Bran
Buckwheat
Bulgar
Couscous
Einkorn
Farro
Freekeh
Grits
Kamut
Kaniwa
Millet
Sorghum
Spelt
Teff
Triticale
Wild Rice

Starch

Chapati
Oatmeal (cooked, unflavored)
Rolled Oats

Vegetables

Acorn squash
Banana Squash
Butternut squash
Cassava
Cherimoya
Delicata Squash
Hubbard Squash
Kabocha
Mamey Sapote (sweet potato like)
Parsnips
Peas
Plantains
Potato
Pumpkin
Sweet Potato
Tamarind
Taro
Yucca root
Yams

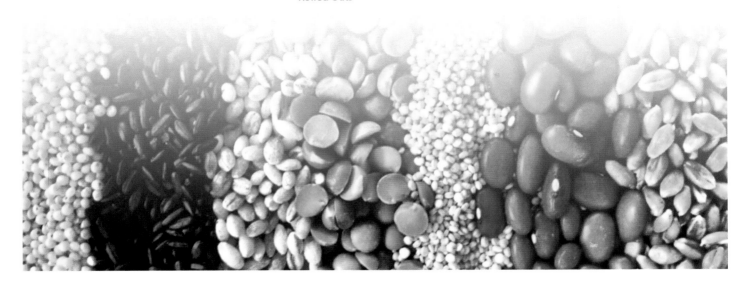

ONLY USE THIS LAYER IF YOUR BLOOD SUGAR FOR TODAY IS UNDER 140

Layer 6: Sparing the Spare Tire. This layer is the lowest layer for your nutrition priorities. It's called sparing the spare tire because having these foods often will add to the spare tire that you're trying to get rid of in the first place. These foods are high in sugar, low in nutrients, and have higher amounts of things that will tend to affect your health. They contain the type of words you've heard of that we want to eat less of like sodium, trans-fats, etc. Also note, any sort of frying will take away from the benefits you want to give yourself. That includes deep fry, shallow fry and such.
This way of eating is not meant to deprive and is based on being realistic. That is why there is still a place for these foods.

Layer 6 (Sparing the Spare Tire)
NOTE: Special Times – pick 2 meals out of the week you want to have this

Beverages

Alcohol
- Beer
- Liquor (all types)
- Wine

Juice
Soda

All Drinks with Sugar Substitutes
Diet Sodas
Sports Drinks
Skim Milk
1% Milk

Fried Foods

French Fries
Hash Browns
Fried Chicken
Fried Egg rolls
Fried Spring rolls
Fried Shrimp
Fried Seafood
Corn Dogs
All Fritters
All Fried Meats

Starch

Bagel
Banana Bread
Bread
Cereals
Chips
Crackers
Croissants
Doughnut
English Muffin
Granola
Hamburger Buns
Hot Dog Buns

Mashed Potatoes
Muffin
Pancake
Pizza
Polenta
Popcorn
Pretzels
Rice Cakes
Taco Shells
Waffle
White Rice
Tortillas (all types)
Taco Shell

Sweets

Bars (all types)
Brownie
Cakes
Candy
Chocolate
Chocolate Covered Foods
Cookies

Cupcake
Frozen Yogurt
Fruit Cobbler
Ice Cream
Jam
Pie
Pudding

Sauces

Alfredo
Amatriciana
Aoili
BBQ (all types - Asian, American, etc.)
Bechamel Sauce
Beurre Manie
Bolognese
Bordelaise Sauce
Buffalo Sauce
Butterscotch
Café de Paris
Caramel Sauce
Carbonara
Cha Siu Sauce
Cocktail Sauce
Coconut Cream
Coulis
Creamy Dressing
Crème Anglaise
Custard
Doenjang
Duck Sauce
Gochujang

Gravy (all types)
Ketchup
Egusi Sauce
Enchilada Sauce
Fudge Sauce
Meuniere Sauce
Mint Sauce
Neopolitan Ragu
Normande Sauce
Peppercorn Sauce
Picadillo
Poutine Sauce
Remoulade
Sambal
Sauce au Poive
Sauce Robert
Sha Cha Sauce
Ssamjang
Steak Sauce
Sweet Bean Sauce (Asian)
Sweet Chili Sauce
Tartar Sauce
Tentsuyu
Teriyaki
XO Sauce

Condiments

Palm Oil
Salad Dressing
Sour Cream
White Sugar

All Dried Fruits

Raisins
Cranberries (Craisins)
Apricots
Bananas
Apples
Pineapple
Mango
Prunes

How to use the LOLS Layers Log (food log).

The LOLS Layers Log is designed as a tool to for you to check off the foods you eat that belong in each of the layers for each meal. If you ate the minimum amount of foods in layers 1, 2, and 3, place a check mark in those respective boxes for each meal. If you did not reach the minimum amount, place an "X" in those boxes. If you did not eat that layer at all, then leave it blank. For the columns labeled 4, 5, and 6, if you ate below the maximum amount for each layer, then place a check mark in those boxes. If you ate above the maximum allowed for each layer, place an "X" in those respective boxes. Do the same for snacks for each layer.

For each meal, to be completely compliant with the plan, you should have at least layers 1, 2, and 3 checked off since they have minimum amounts you have to eat daily. It is totally okay to only eat these layers for the day without touching layers 4, 5, and 6 if your blood sugars are not affected by medications.

In the blood sugar column, make sure to log down your blood sugars BEFORE each meal (if you are told by your physician to check them).

How to analyze the LOLS Layers Log after you use it.

If you look at your daily blood sugars and they are below your goals, then you're doing something right! If you blood sugars are above what you expected, then make sure that for each week, layers 1, 2, and 3 are satisfied with their daily minimums. Then start eliminating layers 5 and/or 6 to see if those will bring down your blood sugars for the following week.

If you are not instructed to check your blood sugars, then visit your physician at the end of 90 days to get your hemoglobin A1C result. If your Hemoglobin A1C is higher than before, then make sure layers 1, 2, and 3 are satisfied with their daily minimums and start eliminating layers 5 and/or 6.

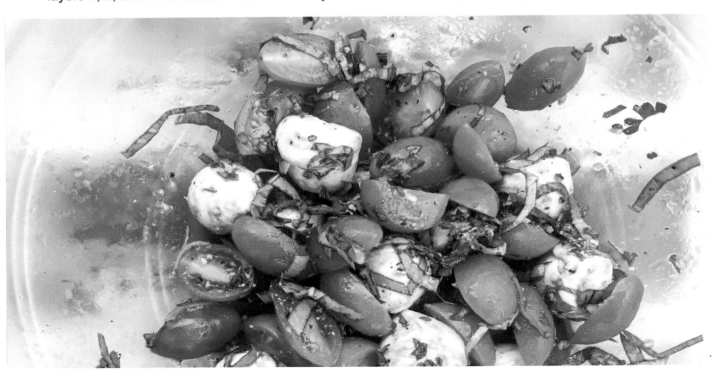

LOLS Layer Log

DustOffDiabetes.com

Name:

Date	Blood Sugar	Layer 1	Layer 2	Layer 3	Layer 4	Layer 5	Layer 6
Monday							
Breakfast							
Lunch							
Dinner							
Snacks							
Tuesday							
Breakfast							
Lunch							
Dinner							
Snacks							
Wednesday							
Breakfast							
Lunch							
Dinner							
Snacks							
Thursday							
Breakfast							
Lunch							
Dinner							
Snacks							
Friday							
Breakfast							
Lunch							
Dinner							
Snacks							
Saturday							
Breakfast							
Lunch							
Dinner							
Snacks							
Sunday							
Breakfast							
Lunch							
Dinner							
Snacks							

Minimums   Maximums   Spare Tire

If your reason is strong enough you will do it.

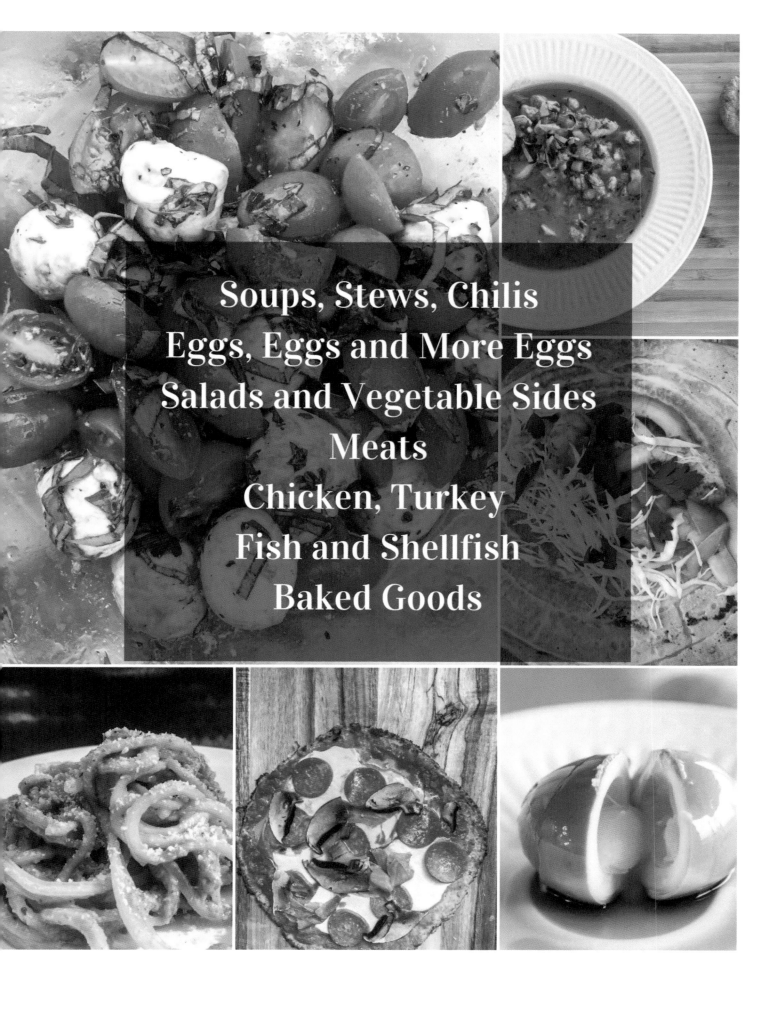

Soups, Stews, Chilis
Eggs, Eggs and More Eggs
Salads and Vegetable Sides
Meats
Chicken, Turkey
Fish and Shellfish
Baked Goods

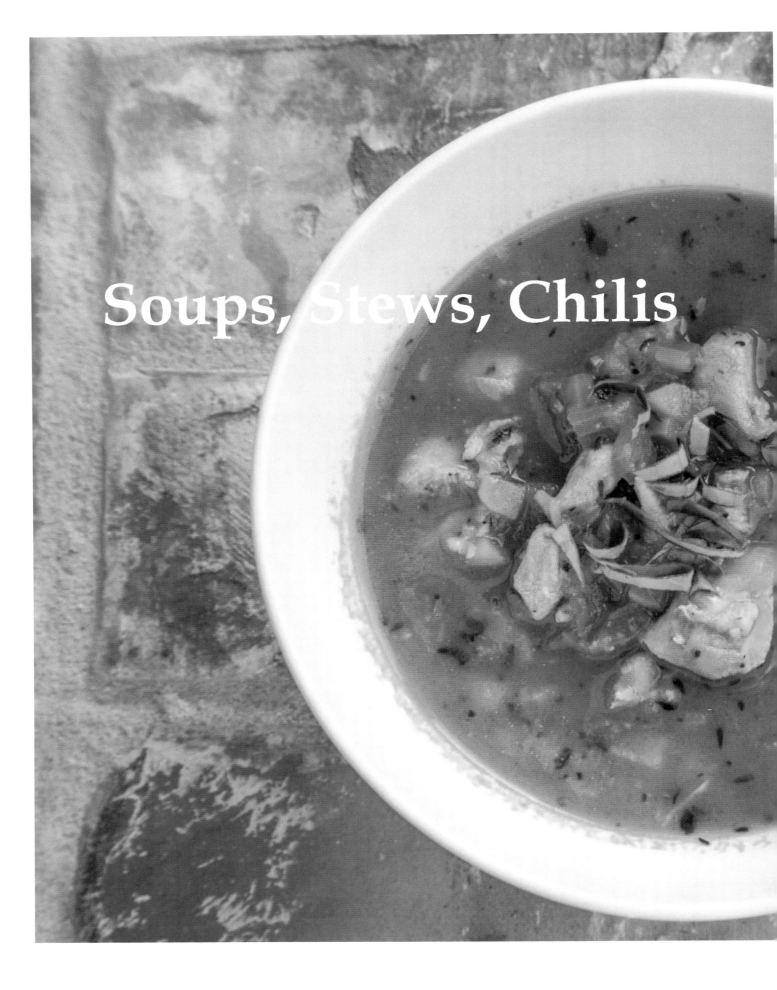

Soups, Stews, Chilis

Hearty Chicken Vegetable Soup

Serves [8]
Prep: 15 minutes
Cook: 45 minutes

3 skinless, boneless chicken thighs (diced)
Kosher salt and pepper
1 teaspoon dried oregano
3 tablespoons olive oil
1 large yellow onion (diced)
¾ pound fresh carrots (diced)
¾ pound fresh celery (diced)
1 teaspoon dried thyme
½ teaspoon black pepper
2 tablespoons tomato paste
2 quarts chicken broth
1 (15-ounce) can of cannellini beans
     (no salt, rinsed and drained)
     -can substitute for aseptic package beans
Kosher salt to taste
Fresh basil, chiffonade (optional)

1. Take the diced chicken thighs and season with salt, pepper and dried oregano. Set aside for use later.

2. Heat a large stock pot over medium heat and add olive oil. Add onion and sauté for 5 minutes until translucent. Add carrots, celery, dried thyme, black pepper and tomato paste. Continue to sauté for 5 minutes until softened.

3. Pour in chicken broth carefully and stir. Add in chicken thighs and drained beans and bring to a boil.

4. Once the soup is at a roaring boil, turn down flame and simmer for 30 minutes.

5. Kosher salt and pepper to taste when done. Garnish with basil and serve.

Note: This soup is very versatile. If you're in the mood to add other green vegetables such as kale, spinach or peas, you can add them during the last 5-10 minutes of simmering time.

Hearty Chicken Vegetable Soup

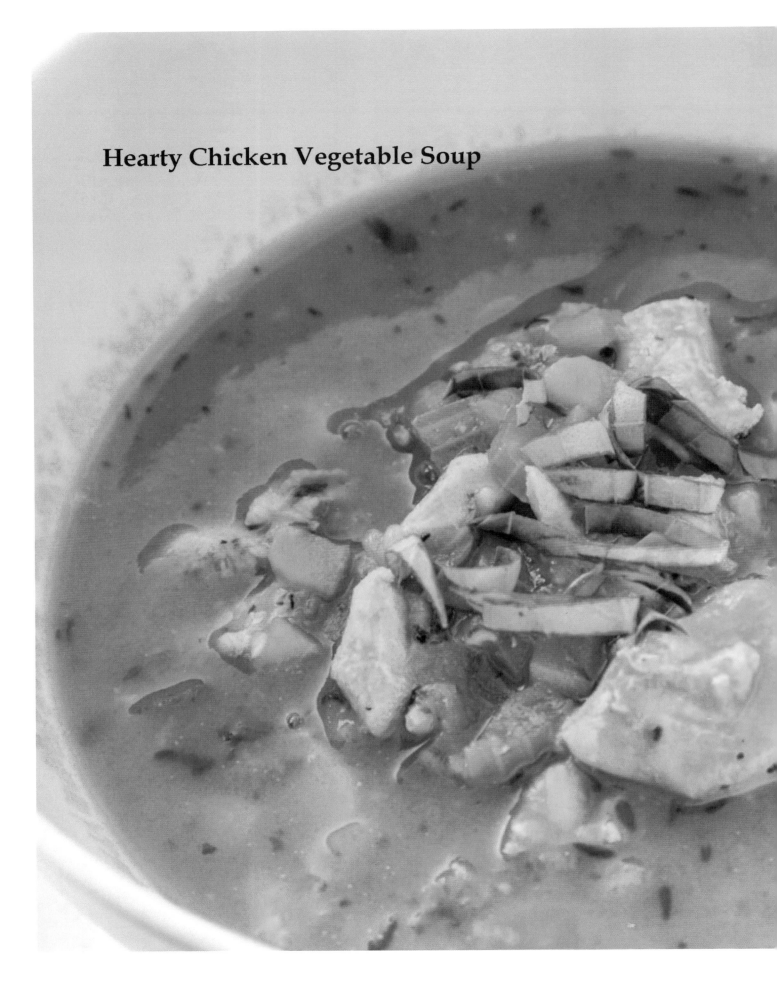

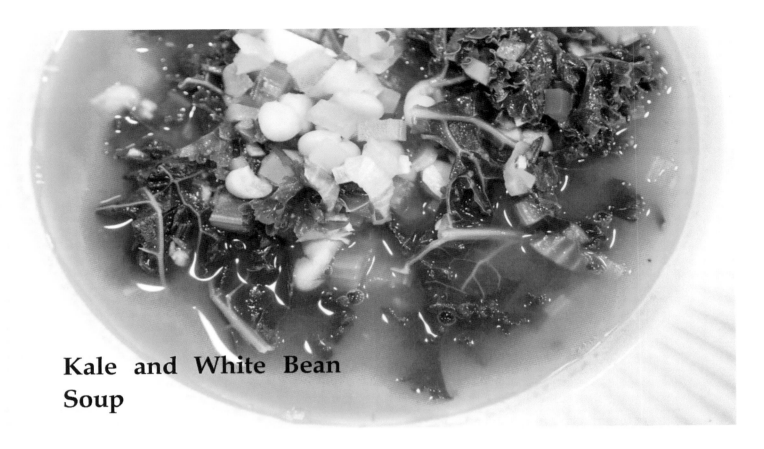

Kale and White Bean Soup

Serves [4]
Prep: 15 minutes
Cook: 20 minutes

3 tablespoons olive oil
1 large yellow onion (diced)
½ pound fresh carrots (diced)
½ pound fresh celery (diced)
2 teaspoon tomato paste
Kosher salt to taste
1 teaspoon ground black pepper
1 quart vegetable broth (preferably organic)
2 (15 ounce) cans of cannellini beans
    (no salt, rinsed and drained)
    -can substitute for aseptic package beans
1 bunch fresh kale leaves (rinsed, drained, bite size)
4 cloves of garlic (minced)
1 teaspoon finely chopped fresh rosemary
1 tablespoon red wine vinegar

1. In a dutch oven over medium heat, add oil and coat the bottom of the pan. Add onion and saute for 2 minutes until translucent. Add carrots, celery, tomato paste, salt and pepper and continue to saute for 5 minutes.

2. Pour vegetable broth into pot. Add beans, kale leaves, garlic and fresh rosemary to soup. Bring to a boil and reduce to a simmer for 5-7minutes.

3. Stir in red wine vinegar. Drizzle with extra virgin olive oil before serving.

Mulligatawny Soup

Serves [8]
Prep: 15 minutes
Cook: 60 minutes

2 tablespoons canola oil
½ cup chopped onions
2 stalks celery, chopped
1 carrot, diced
1 tablespoon butter
1 ¼ tablespoons curry powder
2 quarts of turkey or chicken broth
2 chicken breasts (skinless, boneless, cubed)
½ cup chopped apple
2 cups cauliflower rice
Kosher salt and pepper to taste
½ cup sour cream
¼ cup fresh parsley (chopped)

1. In a large soup pot, add oil and coat the bottom of the pan. Add onions, carrots, celery and butter and saute for 3-5 minutes. Add curry powder and stock. Simmer for about 15 minutes.

2. Add chicken, apple, cauliflower rice and salt and pepper to taste. Simmer for 30 minutes.

3. Stir in sour cream and parsley. Serve immediately.

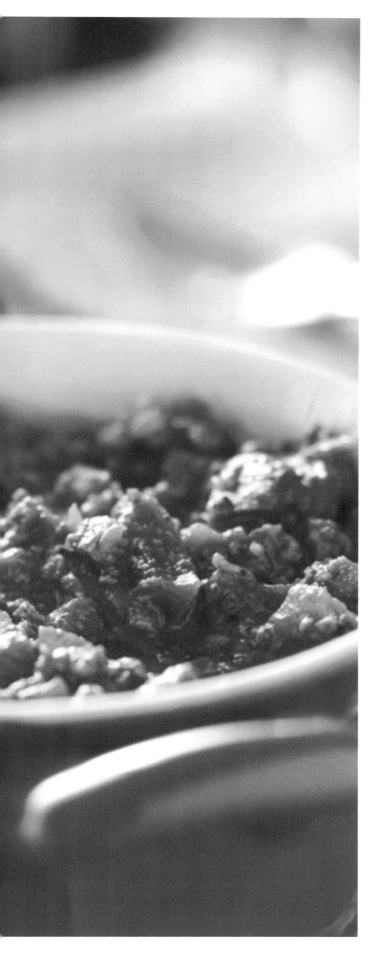

Hearty Beef Stew

Serves [10]
Prep: 25 minutes
Cook: 7 hours

2 pounds beef stew meat
3 tablespoons olive oil
2 cups beef stock
15 oz canned diced tomatoes (drained)
½ cup bell peppers – small dice
½ cup cremini mushrooms (quartered)
¾ cup chopped celery
¾ cup chopped carrot
1 cup chopped onion
1 whole Russet potato (diced)
4 large cloves garlic (minced)
2 tablespoons tomato paste
2 tablespoons Worcestershire Sauce
2 teaspoons Kosher salt
1 ½ teaspoon black pepper
3 sprigs fresh thyme
1 tablespoon chopped fresh parsley

1. Heat slow cooker to low setting.

2. In a large pan over medium high heat, add oil to the heated pan and sear beef on all sides. Transfer beef to the slow cooker.

3. Add stock, tomato, peppers, mushrooms, celery, carrot, onion, garlic, tomato paste, Worcestershire sauce, salt, pepper, and fresh thyme.

4. Cover and cook on low for 7 hours. Add fresh parsley 1 minute before serving and stir to incorporate.

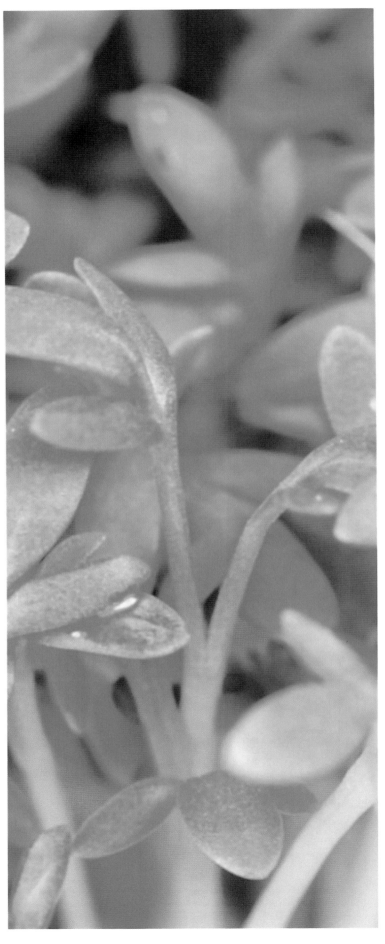

Chinese Watercress with Pork Soup

Serves [4]
Prep: 10 minutes
Cook: 1 hour

½ pound pork butt, cleaned and cut to 1 inch pieces
10 cups of water
10 dried red dates, pitted
1 bunch of fresh watercress, cleaned
Kosher to taste

1. In a medium pot, bring water to a boil and place pork in for 5 minutes. Remove and set aside.

2. In a separate clean pot, pour in water and bring to a boil. Add red dates and pork. Simmer soup 45 minutes.

3. Add watercress to soup and continue to cook for 10 minutes. Season with Kosher salt to taste and serve hot.

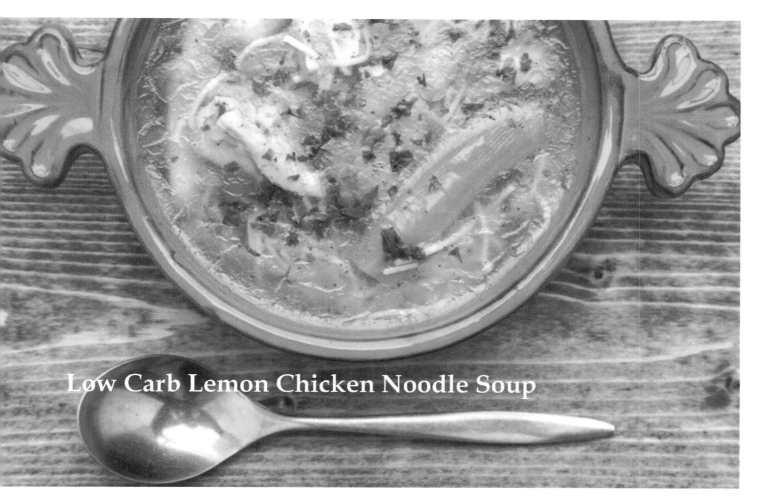

Low Carb Lemon Chicken Noodle Soup

Serves [8]
Prep: 10 minutes
Cook: 20 minutes

3 tablespoons olive oil
1 medium onion (thinly sliced)
8 large cloves garlic (minced)
2 quarts chicken broth
2 whole boneless, skinless chicken breasts
1 large lemon (zested)
½ teaspoon crushed red pepper
Kosher salt and pepper to taste
2 tablespoons feta cheese
¼ cup chopped chives
½ cup chopped carrots
7 oz cooked shirataki noodles

1. In a large pot over medium heat, add oil and coat the bottom of the pan. Add onions and sauté for 5 minutes. Turn heat to low and add garlic. Continue to sauté, careful not to burn garlic.

2. Add stock, chicken, carrot, zest and red pepper to pot. Turn up the heat to high and bring to a boil. Simmer soup after for 10-15 minutes.

3. Add in Shirataki noodles, salt and pepper to taste.

   Remove chicken breast from pot and shred using the chicken using a fork. Pot with feta and chives. Serve hot!

Mexican Chicken Soup with Avocado

Serves [4]
Prep: 10 minutes
Cook: 20 minutes

½ pound chicken breast, boneless
½ teaspoon virgin coconut oil
½ medium yellow onion, diced
1 jalapeno pepper, seeded and minced
2 cloves garlic, minced
2 tomatoes, diced
½ teaspoon cumin
½ teaspoon black pepper
1 teaspoon salt
3 cups chicken broth
1 cup cilantro, chopped
1 avocado, diced
1 lime, juiced
1 lime, cut into wedges (garnish)

1. Clean chicken breast and pat dry. Slice in half length-wise and set aside.

2. In a medium saucepan over medium heat, add coconut oil. Add onion and jalapeño and cook for 2-3 minutes, stirring frequently.

3. Add the garlic and tomatoes to pan and cook for 1 minute. Add cumin, black pepper and salt and stir well to combine. Pour in chicken broth.

4. Add chicken in to soup and bring to a boil. Reduce heat to medium, cover and cook for 10 minutes. Remove chicken from liquid and shred. Return to saucepan and stir in ¾ cup of cilantro (save ¼ cup for garnish)

5. Shred or dice the chicken and return to the saucepan. Stir in ¾ cup of the cilantro (save the rest for garnishing). Add lime juice and stir well.

6. Ladle soup into bowls and add avocado. Garnish with remaining cilantro and lime wedge.

Chicken Vegetable Soup

Serves [6]
Prep: 15 minutes
Cook: 1 hour 40 minutes

2 tablespoons canola oil
1 cup onion, chopped
1 cup celery, chopped
1 cup yellow squash, chopped
2 cups zucchini, chopped
½ cup green beans, chopped
1 pound chicken breast, chopped
1 teaspoon dried basil
1 teaspoon salt
½ teaspoon ground black pepper
1 ½ quart chicken broth

1. In a large pot over medium high heat, add canola oil. Swirl to coat the bottom of pot. Add onion and sauté for 2 minutes. Add celery, yellow squash, zucchini, and green beans and sauté for 2- 3 minutes.

2. Add chicken, basil, black pepper, salt and chicken broth. Bring to a boil and reduce to a simmer, covered, for 1 ½ hours. Serve immediately.

Japanese Inspired Onion Soup

Serves [4]
Prep: 10 minutes
Cook: 45 minutes

1 tablespoon canola oil
2 onions, diced
2 celery stalks, diced
2 carrots, diced
2 cloves garlic, minced
1 ½ quarts vegetable broth
1 teaspoon Kosher salt
½ teaspoon ground black pepper
¼ cup thinly sliced onion
1 cup button mushrooms, thinly sliced
½ cup thinly sliced scallions
Sriracha (optional)

1. In a large pot over medium heat, add canola oil to heated pot. Add diced onions and sauté for 3 minutes until translucent and slightly brown. Add carrots and celery and continue to sauté for 1 minute. Add garlic and continue to cook until fragrant.

2. Pour in vegetable broth and bring to the boil. Add salt and pepper to soup. Lower flame and simmer for 30 minutes.

3. Strain soup and add liquid back to pot. Bring to a boil. Add in sliced onions and simmer for another 10 minutes. Add mushrooms and scallions right before serving. Sriracha seasoning optional.

Low Carb Thai Shrimp Soup

Serves [4]
Prep: 15 minutes
Cook: 25 minutes

2 tablespoons unsalted butter
1 pound medium shrimp, peeled, deveined
Pinch of Kosher salt and freshly ground black pepper
1 tablespoon canola oil
2 cloves garlic, minced
1 medium onion, diced
1 red bell pepper, diced
1 tablespoon freshly grated ginger
2 tablespoons red curry paste
24 ounces unsweetened coconut milk
1 quart vegetable stock
1 cup cooked cauliflower rice
Juice of 1 lime
2 tablespoons fresh chopped cilantro

1. In a large stockpot over medium high heat, melt butter and add shrimp. Season with a pinch of salt and ground black pepper and sauté for 2 minutes until pink. Set aside.

2. In same pot over medium high heat, top with canola oil and add garlic, onion and bell pepper to the stockpot.

   Cook for 3 minutes, continually stirring. Add ginger and continue to stir until fragrant.

3. Add curry paste to pot and stir until well combined. Cook for 1 minute until all ingredients are coated. Whisk in coconut milk and vegetable stock, and cook for 2 minutes. Bring soup to a boil and reduce heat to simmer for 10 minutes.

4. Add shrimp, cauliflower rice, lime juice and cilantro. Cook for 1 minute and serve immediately.

Tuscan White Bean Kale and Sausage Soup

Serves [8]
Prep: 15 minutes
Cook: 50 minutes

1 tablespoon olive oil
12 ounces kielbasa sausage, ¼ inch slices
1 medium onion, diced
3 carrots, diced
2 celery stalks, diced
4 cloves garlic, minced
4 ½ cups chicken stock
2 cups water
1 tablespoon dried parsley
1 teaspoon dried rosemary, crushed
½ teaspoon dried oregano
1 teaspoon Kosher salt
¼ teaspoon freshly ground black pepper
3 cups chopped kale, ribs removed
2 (13.5 ounces) cans cannellini beans, drained and rinsed
Extra Virgin Olive Oil
Shredded parmesan cheese

1. In a large stock pot over medium heat, add olive oil and sausage. Cook for 5 minutes until slightly browned on both sides.

2. Remove sausage and set aside on paper towels to absorb some oil.

3. In same pot over medium heat, add onion, carrots, celery and sauté for 5 minutes. Add garlic and continue to sauté for 1 minute.

4. Add stock, water, parsley, rosemary, oregano, salt and pepper. Bring to a boil and continue to cook for 15 minutes.

5. Add kale and cannellini beans and allow to boil 10 minutes more.

6. Stir in cooked sausage. Drizzle with extra virgin olive oil, top with shredded parmesan and serve forth.

Wake up in the morning and do something for yourself for 5 minutes. Those 5 minutes of positive attitude initiation with make your entire day brighter no matter what you're doing.

Dr. Cheng Ruan

Low Carb Thai Chicken Zoodle Soup

Serves [8]
Prep: 10 minutes
Cook: 30 minutes

1 whole zucchini
1 tablespoon coconut oil
½ red onion, diced
1 jalapeño, small dice
2 cloves garlic, minced
1 ½ tablespoon green curry paste
1 ½ quarts chicken broth
1 (15 ounces) can coconut milk
1 red pepper, julienned
1 pound chicken thigh, skinless, boneless, thinly sliced
2 tablespoons fish sauce
½ cup chopped cilantro
Lime wedges

1. Using a spiralizer, spiralizer zucchini into zoodles. Place zoodles onto paper towels to absorb moisture and set aside.

2. In a large pot over medium heat, heat coconut oil until melted. Add onions and sauté for 5 minutes until translucent.

3. Combine jalapeño and garlic in pot. Add curry paste and sauté for 1 minute.

4. Add chicken broth and stir well. Whisk coconut milk into soup until incorporated. Bring soup to a boil and reduce heat to medium.

5. Add red pepper, chicken and fish sauce. Cook for 5-10 minutes. Stir in chopped cilantro.

6. Divide zoodles into 4 soup bowls and ladle soup over zoodles. Let sit for 2 minutes. Serve with lime wedges.

Sometimes we need to do things for ourselves. Take 5 minutes out of the day and be happy on purpose.

Dr. Cheng Ruan

Creamy Zucchini Soup

Serves [2]
Prep: 10 minutes
Cook: 20 minutes

1 tablespoon olive oil
2 cloves garlic, crushed
3 zucchini, trimmed, chopped
½ teaspoon salt
¼ teaspoon fresh ground black pepper
2 cups chicken broth
1 cup fresh basil leaves
½ cup heavy cream

1. In a large pot over medium heat, add olive oil and garlic. Sauté for 1 minute until fragrant (watch not to burn garlic).

2. Add zucchini, salt, and pepper to pot and cook for 5 minutes until zucchini is tender.

3. Pour in chicken broth and bring to a boil. Let simmer for 10 minutes. Add basil leaves and remove from heat. Let sit for 2 minutes.

4. Transfer soup to blender or use a handheld blender in pot. Blend until smooth. Return to pot and add heavy cream. Stir well to incorporate and serve forth. Drizzle with more cream as garnish

When it comes to food addiction, all it takes is once taste. That's why eating in moderation doesn't work. It's like me telling a cocaine addict to cut down to one line a day instead of 4. In the end, they are still using the same thing as their reward.

Dr. Cheng Ruan

Paleo Seafood Chowder

Serves [8]
Prep: 20 minutes
Cook: 1 hour

½ pound calamari, cut into ½ inch pieces
Juice of 1 lemon
3 tablespoons extra virgin coconut oil
1 medium onion, diced
4 cloves garlic, minced
2 cups carrots, chopped
2 cups celery, chopped
1 quart seafood broth
2 cups water
1 cup tomato sauce
Kosher salt and ground
black pepper to taste
1 teaspoon dried basil
2 teaspoon dried oregano
1 teaspoon dried thyme
1 teaspoon fresh dill
2 teaspoons red pepper flakes
3 whole bay leaves
1 cup chopped mushrooms
½ cup coconut cream
½ pound fresh cod, cleaned
½ pound shrimp, peeled, deveined
1 tablespoon fresh basil, chopped
Lime wedge
Chopped fresh parsley (garnish)

1. Take cut calamari and soak in lemon juice. Set aside.

2. In a large soup pot over medium flame, heat up 3 tablespoons coconut oil and swirl to coat bottom of pot. Add diced onion and sauté for 2 minutes. Add garlic, stir to make sure garlic doesn't burn.

3. Add carrots and celery to pot and continue to cook for 3 minutes, stirring constantly.

4. Pour in broth, water and tomato sauce. Add salt, pepper, dried basil, oregano, thyme, dill, pepper flakes, and bay leaves to soup. Bring to a boil and then simmer for 30 minutes.

5. After 30 minutes, add chopped mushrooms and coconut cream. Bring back to a boil and turn down flame to simmer. Add in cod and cook for 10 minutes. Break apart fish into bite size pieces in soup.

6. Add shrimp and calamari to soup and let cook for 3-5 minutes. Remove bay leaves from soup prior to serving.

7. Serve hot with lime wedges and garnished with parsley.

Beef and Quinoa Soup

Serves [6]
Prep: 30 minutes
Cook: 8 hours

1 ½ pounds beef chuck
Kosher salt and ground black pepper
2 tablespoons olive oil
1 quart beef stock
1 cup celery, chopped
1 cup carrot, chopped
½ cup onion, chopp
1 whole roma tomato, diced
3 cloves garlic, minced
½ cup quinoa, rinsed
2 tablespoons Worcestershire sauce
1 teaspoon Kosher salt
½ teaspoon fresh ground black pepper

1. Heat slow cooker on low setting.

2. Pat beef chuck dry and season with salt and pepper. In a large pan over medium high heat, add olive oil and sear beef on both sides until browned. Remove from pan and let rest for 5 minutes. Cut into 1 inch chunks and add to slow cooker.

3. Pour beef stock into slow cooker. Add celery, carrot, onion, tomato, minced garlic, quinoa, Worcestershire sauce, sea salt and black pepper. Cover and cook for 8 hours on low setting.

Toxins can enter your body through breathing and through your mouth. You can control only one of those right now.

Dr. Cheng Ruan

Sweet Potato Cauliflower Sausage Soup

Serves [8]
Prep: 15 minutes
Cook: 1 hours 15 minutes

6 cups cauliflower florets
1 tablespoons olive oil
Kosher salt and black pepper
1 tablespoon olive oil
1 pound spicy Italian sausage, casing removed
1 tablespoon olive oil
1 whole medium onion, diced
2 whole leeks, cleaned, thinly sliced
2 tablespoons minced garlic
2 teaspoons garlic powder
1 teaspoon Kosher salt
1 teaspoon ground black pepper
1 ½ quart chicken stock
½ pound sweet potato, diced
1 cup cremini mushrooms, quartered
1 ½ cups fresh baby spinach leaves

1. Preheat oven to 400°F. In a large bowl, toss cauliflower florets with olive oil, season with salt and pepper. On a sheet pan lined with parchment paper, place cauliflower evenly spaced and roast for 30 minutes until slightly brown.

2. In a large pot over medium high heat, add oil and Italian sausage. Use spatula to break up sausage into bite size pieces while browning. Set aside.

3. In same pot, lower heat to medium, add olive oil, onion and leeks. Sauté for 5-10 minutes.

4. Add garlic and stir for 1 minute until fragrant. Add roasted cauliflower, garlic powder, salt and pepper. Pour chicken stock and bring to a boil. Reduce heat and simmer for 10 minutes.

5. Transfer soup to a blender (work in batches if all the soup cannot fit into one blender). Blend until smooth.

6. Return soup to pot and bring back to a boil. Add cooked sausage, sweet potato, cremini mushrooms to pot. Cook for 10 minutes or until potato is tender.

Stir in spinach leaves and continue to cook for 2 minutes. Serve immediately.

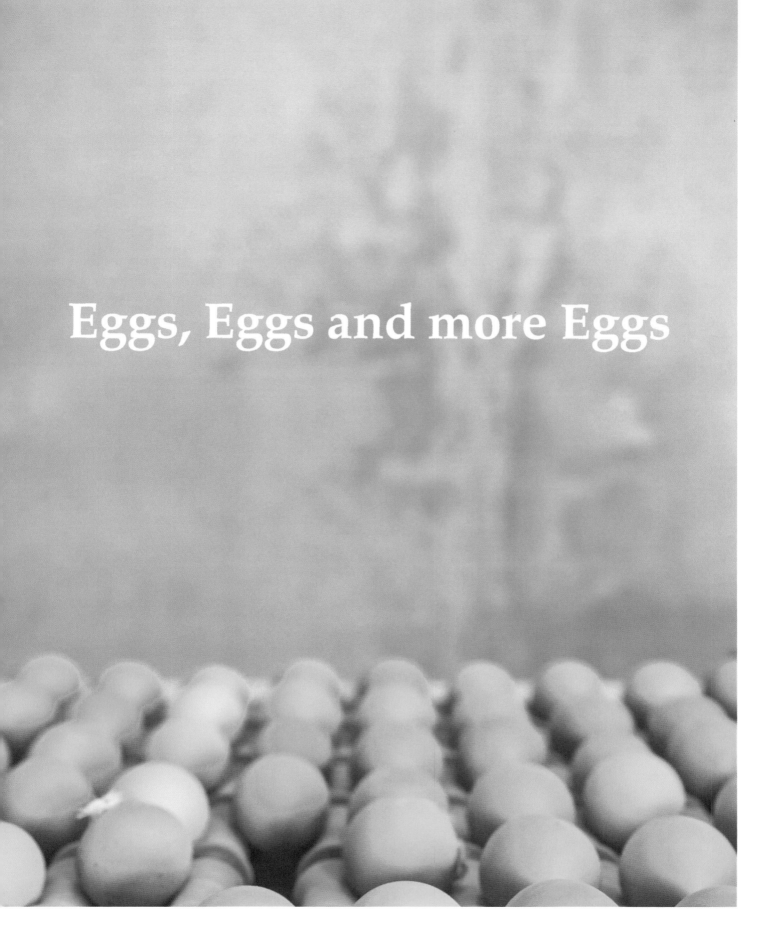

Eggs, Eggs and more Eggs

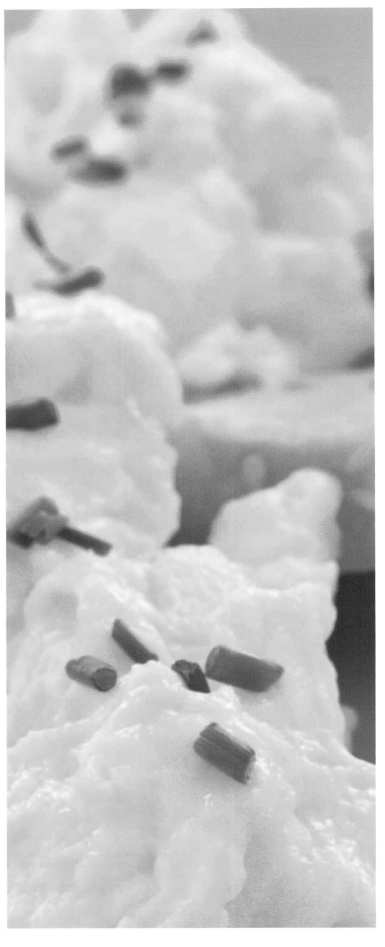

Simple Scrambled Eggs

Serves [1]
Prep: 5 minutes
Cook: 1 minutes

2 whole extra large eggs
2 tablespoons whole milk
Dash of Kosher salt and pepper
1 teaspoon canola oil

1. Crack eggs into a large bowl. Add milk, salt and pepper to taste. Whisk until incorporated and set aside.

2. In a large nonstick pan over medium heat, heat up canola oil and pour in egg mixture. Using a spatula, constantly stir eggs until there's no more liquid in the pan, approximately 1-2 minutes.

3. Remove from heat and serve immediately.

Perfect Hard Boiled Eggs

Prep: 5 minutes
Cook: 8 minutes

6 large eggs (preferably organic)

1. In a 2 quart pot, fill halfway with cold water. Rinse eggs and place into pot.

2. Cover and bring to a boil. Remove from heat once the water is a roaring boil. Let it sit for 8 minutes.

3. Prepare an ice bath in the meantime. Drain and place eggs into ice bath. This should stop the cooking process. Store in an airtight container for up to 4 days.

Perfect Soft Boiled Eggs

Prep: 5 minutes
Cook: 8 minutes

6 large eggs (preferably organic)

1. In a 2 quart pot, fill halfway with cold water. Rinse eggs and place into pot.

2. Cover and bring to a boil. Remove from heat once the water is a roaring boil. Let it sit for 4 minutes.

3. Prepare an ice bath in the meantime. Drain and place eggs into ice bath. This should stop the cooking process. Store in an airtight container for up to 2 days.

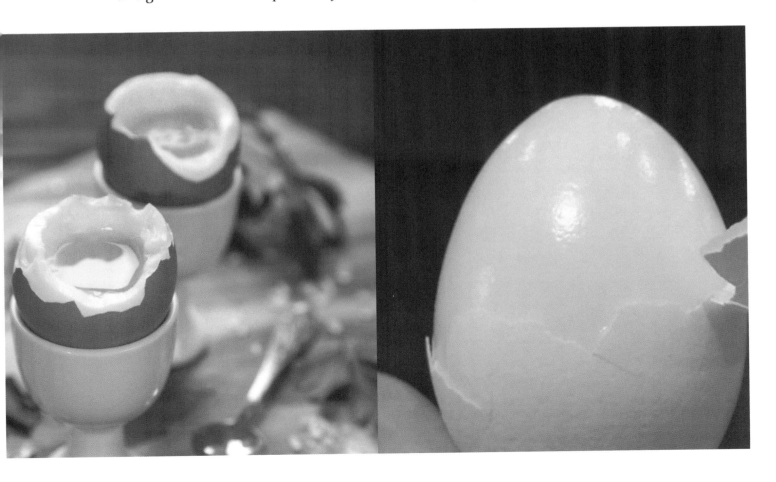

Tarragon Soft Scrambled Eggs

Serves [1]
Prep: 5 minutes
Cook: 1 minutes

2 whole extra large eggs
1 tablespoon whole milk
½ teaspoon dried tarragon
Dash of Kosher salt and pepper
1 teaspoon canola oil

1. Crack eggs into a large bowl. Add milk, tarragon, salt and pepper to taste. Whisk until incorporated and set aside.

2. In a large nonstick pan over medium heat, heat up canola oil and pour in egg mixture. Using a spatula, constantly stir eggs until there's no more liquid in the pan, usually 30 seconds to 1 minute.

3. Remove from heat and serve immediately.

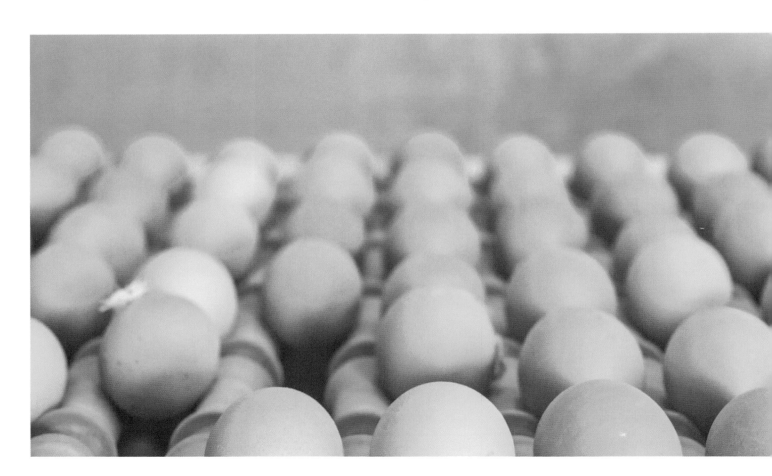

Shoyu Tamgo (Soy Sauce Eggs)

Serves [6]
Prep: 10 minutes
Cook: 4-6 hours for marination

½ cup warm water
1 tablespoon cane sugar
¾ cup low-sodium soy sauce
2 tablespoons red wine vinegar
2 tablespoons mirin
6 large eggs

1. Combine water, sugar, soy sauce, vinegar and mirin in a bowl and whisk until sugar is dissolved. Pour mixture into a sealable container and set aside.

2. Bring a large pot of water to a boil. Using a wire mesh or slotted spoon, slowly lower the eggs into water and stir for 2 minutes, continue to cook for another 5 minutes for a total of 7 minutes. Place eggs into ice bath. Crack eggs and slowly peel the shell off. It will still be very delicate.

3. Place eggs carefully into the marinade and place two pieces of paper towels into the marinade over the eggs, until saturated with soy sauce mixture. This will help keep the eggs from floating to the top. Marinate in the fridge for 4-6 hours. Remove eggs and store in airtight container for up to 1 week.

4. Cut lengthwise prior to serving. The egg white should be firm while the yolk is slightly runny.

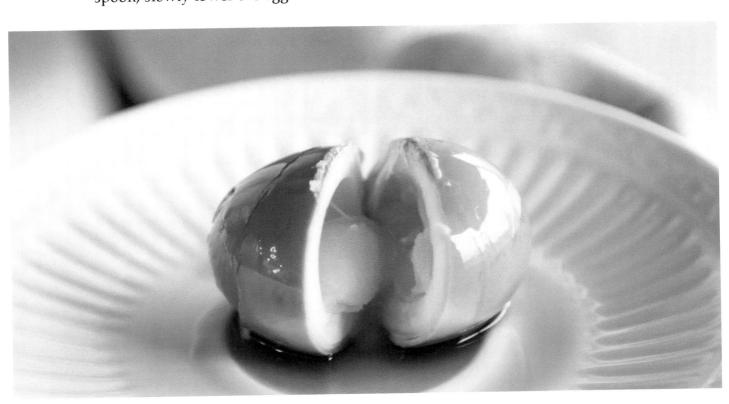

Crust-less Broccoli Cheddar Quiche

Serves [6]
Prep: 15 minutes
Cook: 40 minutes

Butter to coat muffin tin
Kosher salt
3 cups small broccoli florets
1 teaspoon canola oil
1 cup yellow onion (diced)
8 large eggs
1 cup whole milk
⅔ cup heavy cream
Nutmeg
4oz cheddar cheese (shredded)
1 tablespoon fresh parsley (chopped)
Kosher salt and pepper to taste

1. Preheat oven to 350°F and set rack to the middle of the oven. Grease 12 cup muffin pan and set aside.

2. Bring a large pot of water to a boil over high heat and add salt. Add in broccoli and gently stir for 1 minute. Drain and set aside.

3. In a medium nonstick skillet, heat up canola oil over medium heat and add diced onions. Sauté for 2 minutes or until translucent. Set aside.

4. In a large mixing bowl, whisk together eggs, whole milk, heavy cream, nutmeg, salt and pepper. Stir in broccoli, onion, cheese and fresh parsley.

5. Ladle mixture into muffin cup, filling ¾ of the way. Your quiche will need room to expand.

6. Bake for 35-40 minutes or until the custard is set in the center. Remove and cool slightly before serving.

Note: This can be prepared in large batches ahead of time and frozen for easy snacks or meals on the fly. Great for breakfast, lunch or dinner.

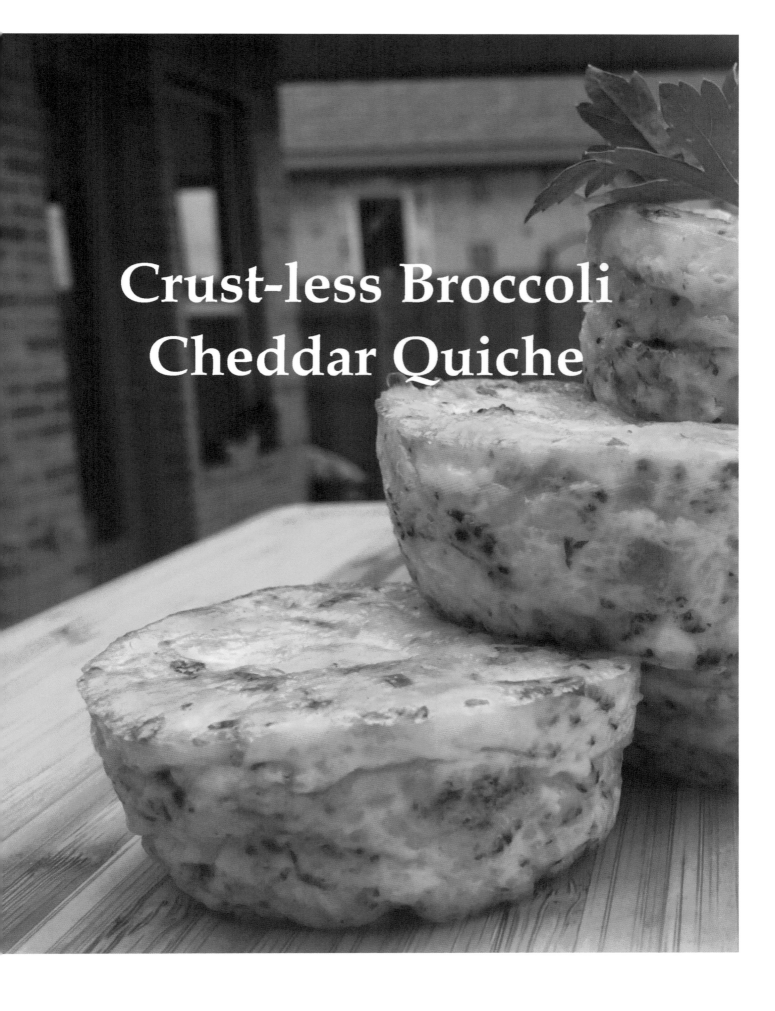

Crust-less Broccoli Cheddar Quiche

Savory Steamed Egg Custard

Serves [2]
Prep: 10 minutes
Cook: 25 minutes

5 whole dried shrimps
4 large eggs
1 cup chicken stock (or water)
Pinch of Kosher Salt
¼ teaspoon ground white pepper
½ teaspoon sesame oil
Seasoned soy sauce (optional)
Scallion, thinly sliced greens only (garnish)

1. Rinse dried shrimps and soak in water for 5 minutes.

2. Whisk eggs in a large bowl. Add stock, pinch of salt, pepper and sesame oil and continue to whisk until smooth. Strain mixture through a fine sieve into a heat proof dish. Take dried shrimps out of soaking liquid and mince. Sprinkle into egg mixture.

3. In a large pot, add enough water to reach steamer and bring to a gentle boil (avoid high heat for a smooth texture). Gently lower egg dish into the steamer. Cover and steam for 20 minutes.

4. Carefully remove dish from steamer. Drizzle with soy sauce and garnish with scallion. Serve immediately.

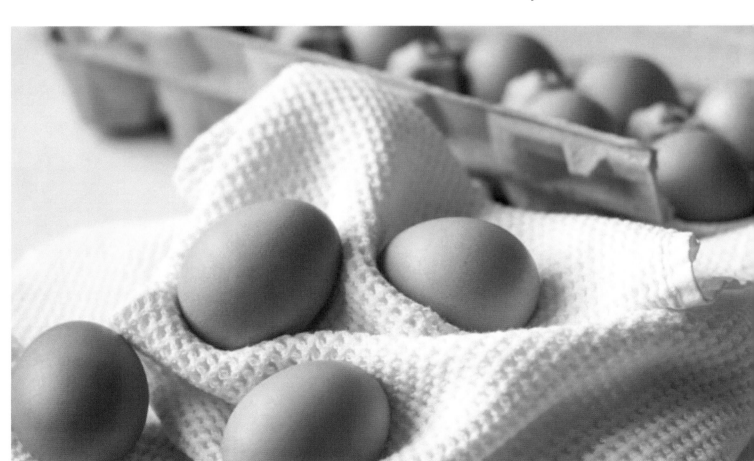

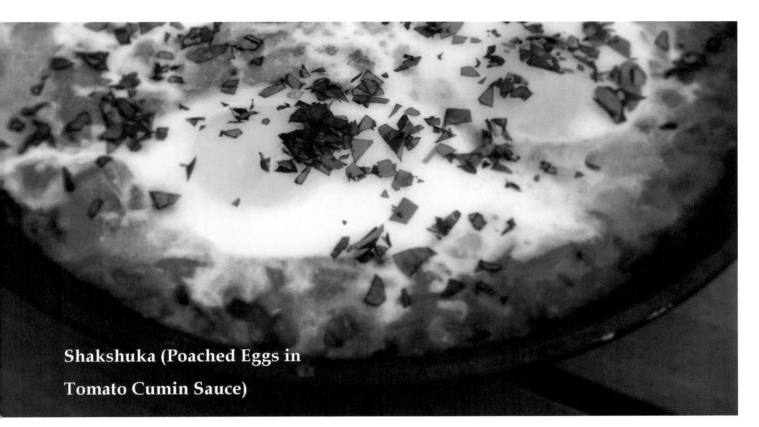

Shakshuka (Poached Eggs in Tomato Cumin Sauce)

Serves [3-4]
Prep: 10 minutes
Cook: 40 minutes

3 tablespoons olive oil
1 large onion, thinly sliced
1 large bell pepper, seeded, julienned
6 garlic cloves, thinly sliced
1 teaspoon cumin
1 teaspoon paprika
⅛ teaspoon cayenne pepper
1 tablespoon tomato paste
1 (28-ounce) can whole plum tomatoes (rough chopped) or 4 cups of ripe tomatoes (diced)
Kosher salt and pepper to taste
6 large eggs
Fresh cilantro, chopped (garnish)

1. In a large skillet over medium heat, add olive oil onion and bell pepper and saute for 10 minutes until soften. Add garlic, cumin, paprika, cayenne pepper and tomato paste and cook for 2 minutes.

2. Pour in tomatoes, salt and pepper and simmer for 15-20 minutes, until sauce thickens.

3. Gently crack eggs over tomato sauce in skillet and cover for 5 minutes. The whites should be set while the yolk maintains a runny texture. If you like the yolk firmer, cover for 7-8 minutes. Add water to the sauce if it's a little dry.

4. Garnish with cilantro and serve forth.

Artichoke Leek Frittata

Serves [4]
Prep: 20 minutes
Cook: 35 minutes

1 tablespoon butter
2 cups leeks, cleaned and sliced
½ cup artichoke hearts sliced
½ teaspoon dried tarragon
¼ teaspoon Kosher salt
5 eggs
1 cup ricotta cheese
½ teaspoon baking powder
1 cup grated Parmesan cheese
1 tablespoon butter
1 tablespoon fresh parsley, chopped

1. In a medium oven safe pan, melt butter over medium heat and add the sliced leeks. Cook for 8-10 minutes until softened. Add the artichoke hearts, tarragon, and salt. Cook for 5 minutes and set mixture aside in a bowl.

2. In a separate bowl, whisk eggs and ricotta cheese together. In another bowl, combine flour, Parmesan, baking powder and whisk to incorporate. Slowly add the dry ingredients to the egg mixture and whisk to combine. Stir in the artichoke and leeks.

3. Wipe down your pan and melt butter in the pan over medium heat, making sure the bottom is coated. Pour in egg mixture and spread mixture until even. Turn down heat to low and cover. Cook for 15 minutes, or until eggs isset except for center.

4. Preheat the broiler. Broil for 3-4 minutes until center is set and color is golden brown.

5. Remove from oven and use a spatula to loosen frittata from pan. Gently slide onto serving plate and garnish with parsley before serving.

Tex-Mex Scramble Eggs

Serves [2]
Prep: 20 minutes
Cook: 35 minutes

1 tablespoon coconut oil
5 extra large eggs
2 tablespoons chopped green bell pepper
2 tablespoons diced red onion
3 cherry tomatoes, diced
¼ cup frozen spinach, drained
2 jalapeños, seeded and diced
¼ cup shredded cheddar cheese
2 tablespoons salsa

1. In a large non-stick pan over medium heat, add coconut oil.

2. In a large bowl, combine eggs, pepper, onion, tomatoes, spinach and jalepeno. Whisk until incorporated well.

3. Pour the mixture into the skillet, making sure the mixture is even in the pan. Cook for 3-5 minutes.

4. Add cheese right before eggs are done and let it melt.

5. Garnish with salsa on top and serve forth.

Setting goals and tracking your progress is the most underutilized tool for success.

Dr. Cheng Ruan

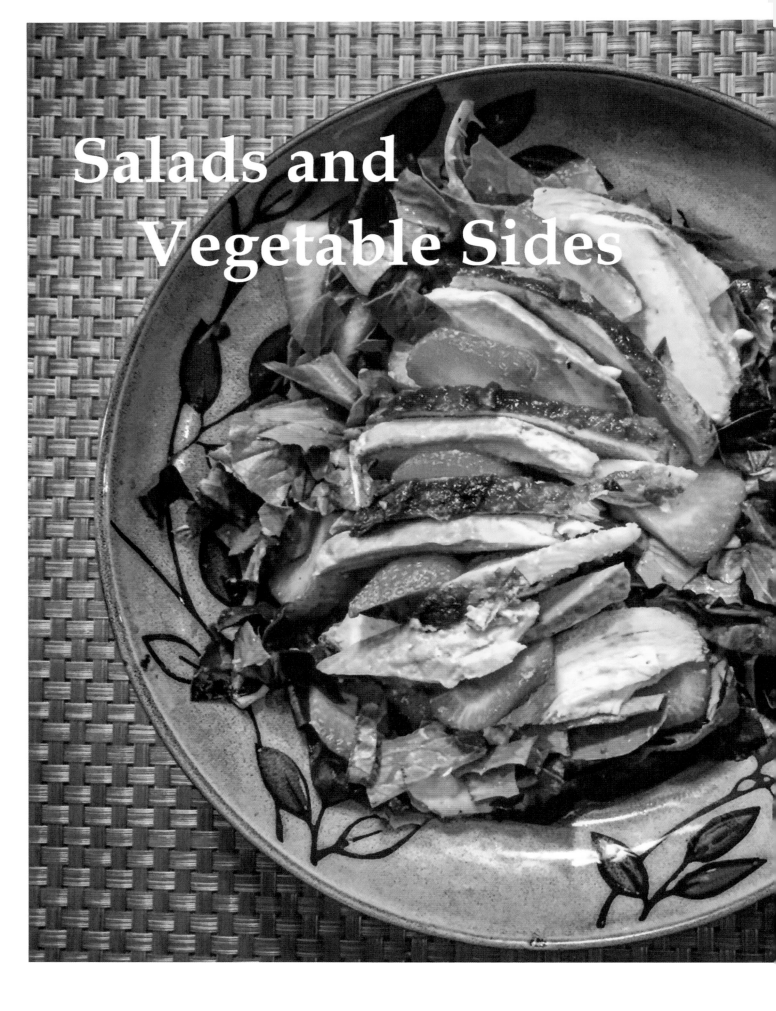

Salads and
Vegetable Sides

Roasted Brussel Sprouts with Lemon Zest

Serves [2]
Prep: 5 minutes
Cook: 40 minutes

8 ounces fresh Brussel sprouts
2 tablespoon canola oil
¼ teaspoon ground black pepper
Kosher salt to taste
Zest of 1 lemon

1. Preheat oven to 400°F.

2. In a large bowl, toss cleaned Brussel sprouts with oil, salt and fresh black pepper until coated.

3. On a lined sheet pan with parchment paper, spread Brussel sprouts onto sheet pan making sure not to crowd the pan. Roast for 35-40 minutes or until crisp on the outside.

4. Sprinkle evenly with lemon zest and serve immediately.

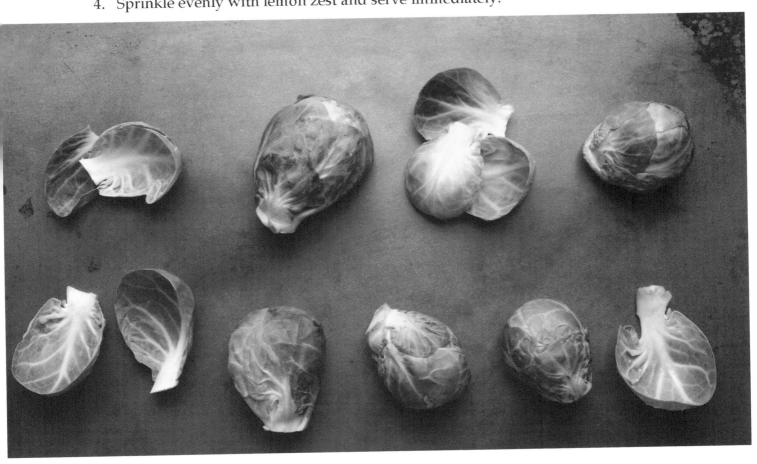

Mushroom Fricassee

Serves [4]
Prep: 10 minutes
Cook: 15 minutes

½ cup beef or chicken broth
2 tablespoons olive oil
1 tablespoon butter (preferably grass fed)
2 cloves garlic (sliced)
1 shallot (finely chopped)
½ pound crimini mushrooms caps (cleaned and sliced)
½ pound oyster mushrooms (cleaned and sliced)
¼ teaspoon ground black pepper
Kosher salt to taste
2 tablespoons balsamic vinegar
Coarsely chopped parsley (garnish)

1. In a large nonstick skillet on medium high heat, add olive oil, butter and add garlic and shallots. Stir for a few seconds until softened.

2. Add mushrooms, black pepper and salt to taste to skillet. Pour stock and cook for 7-10 minutes, stirring constantly. Add balsalmic vinegar and continue to cook for 1-2 minutes.

3. Garnish with parsley before serving.

When it comes to food addiction, all it takes is once taste. That's why eating in moderation doesn't work. It's like me telling a cocaine addict to cut down to one line a day instead of 4. In the end, they are still using the same thing as their reward.

Dr. Cheng Ruan

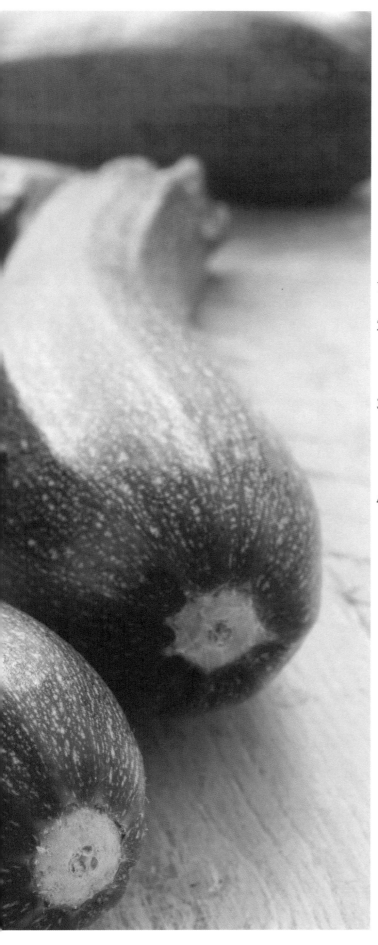

Zucchini Chips

Prep: 15 minutes
Cook: 2-3 hours

4 cups thinly sliced zucchini (practically paper thin)
2 tablespoon olive oil
Kosher salt to taste

1. Preheat oven to 225°F.

2. Take zucchini slices and pat with paper towel to try out some moisture. Place all into a bowl and toss with olive oil.

3. On a lined sheet pan, place each slice of zucchini next to each other. Do not overlap the slices. Sprinkle with Kosher salt.

4. Bake for 2-3 hours until golden and crisp. Remove and let it cool before serving.

Sautéed Broccoli Rabe

Prep: 5 minutes
Cook: 10 minutes

1 bunch broccoli rabe (cleaned)
2 tablespoon olive oil
3 cloves garlic, crushed
½ teaspoon crushed red pepper
Kosher salt and pepper to taste

1. Bring a large pot of water to boil and blanch broccoli rabe for 1 minute. Remove and add to a bowl of ice water to stop cook process.

2. In a large pan over medium heat, add garlic and red pepper flakes and sauté for 1-2 minutes. Discard garlic cloves and add broccoli rabe into pan.

3. Continue to sauté for 5-7 minutes and season to taste.

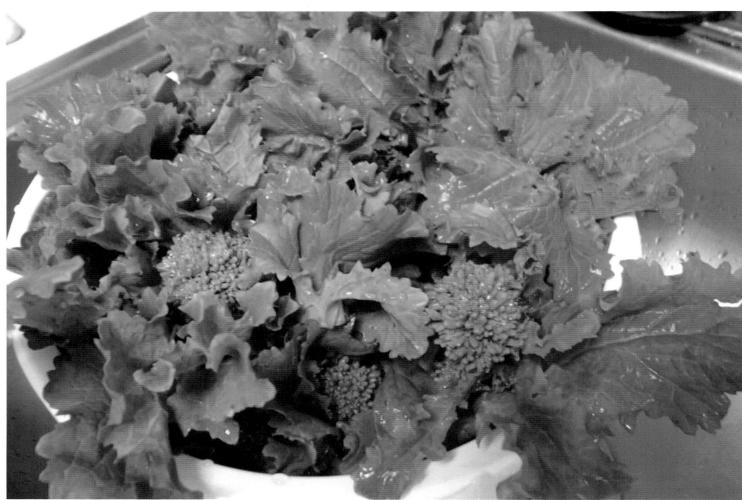

Roasted Spaghetti Squash and Meatballs

Serves [8]
Prep: 20 minutes
Cook: 1 hour

1 large spaghetti squash
1 tablespoon olive oil (for brushing)
1 pound grass fed ground beef
1 onion, finely diced
1 extra large egg
1 tablespoon Pecorino Romano cheese, grated
1 tablespoon ground cumin
1 teaspoon paprika
1 teaspoon dried thyme
2 teaspoons Kosher salt
1 teaspoon ground black pepper
4 tablespoons sesame oil
6 slices fresh mozzarella
1 cup Rao's Homemade Marinara Sauce
1 bunch fresh parsley leaves, chopped
Ground black pepper to taste

To make spaghetti squash:

1. Preheat oven to 400°F. Slice spaghetti squash in half. Remove seeds and brush inside with olive oil.

2. Place onto lined baking sheet and roast for 35 minutes.

3. Remove and shred squash with a fork until it has the appearance of long strands of spaghetti.

4. Pour marinara sauce evenly into two halves of squash, top with mozzarellas slices.

5. Place back in oven to cook at 500°F for 10 minutes. Garnish with parsley and black pepper to taste.

To make meatballs and assembly:

1. In a large bowl, mix beef with onion, egg, grated cheese, cumin, paprika, thyme, salt and pepper.

2. Form into balls with your hands.

3. Preheat oven to 450°F. In an oven safe large frying pan over medium high heat, add sesame oil. Sear meatballs until browned on all sides. Place in oven and cook for 10 minutes.

4. Place meatballs on top of cooked spaghetti squash and serve hot.

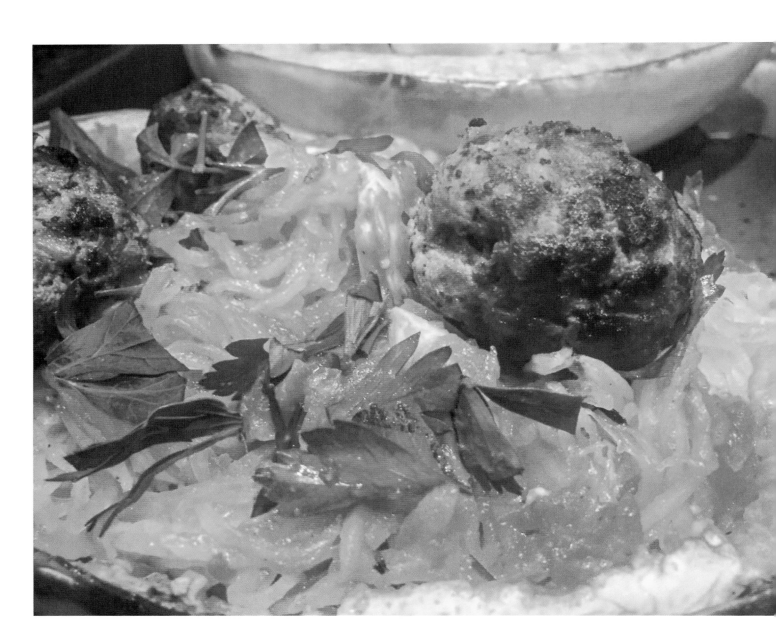

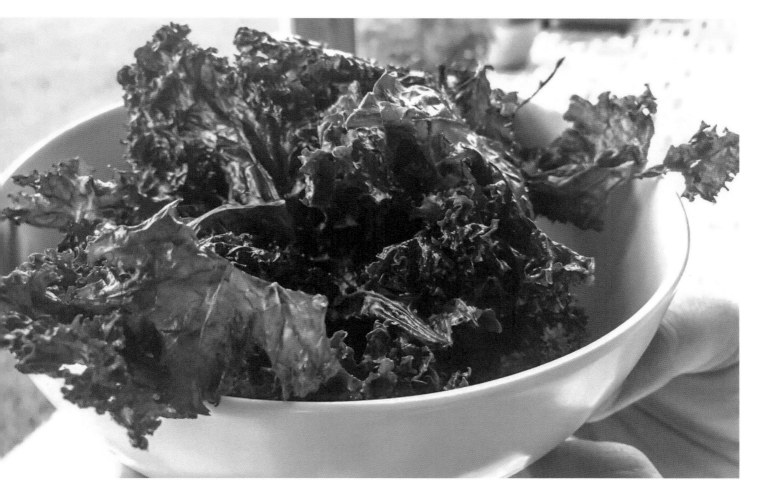

Kale Chips

Prep: 5 minutes
Cook: 25 minutes

1 bunch kale (cleaned, trimmed, leaves only)
2 tablespoon olive oil
Kosher salt and ground black pepper to coat
½ cup nutritional yeast (optional)

1. Preheat oven to 350°F.

2. Pat kale leaves dry and make sure to cut 2 inch pieces. In a large bowl, add kale, olive oil, and nutritional yeast. Toss to coat well.

3. Line 2 baking sheets with parchment paper and arrange kale on a single layer. Sprinkle with Kosher salt and pepper. Make sure not to crowd the pan or it will steam instead of crisp.

4. Bake for 25-30 minutes, until crisp.

Caprese Salad

Prep: 10 minutes

1 cup red cherry tomatoes, cut in half
1 cup yellow cherry tomatoes, cut in half
1 cup fresh mozzarella balls
¼ cup chopped fresh parsley
2 tablespoons chopped fresh basil
Kosher salt and pepper to taste

1. In a large tossing bowl, add cherry tomatoes, fresh mozzarella, parsley basil and salt. Gently toss and season with ground black pepper.

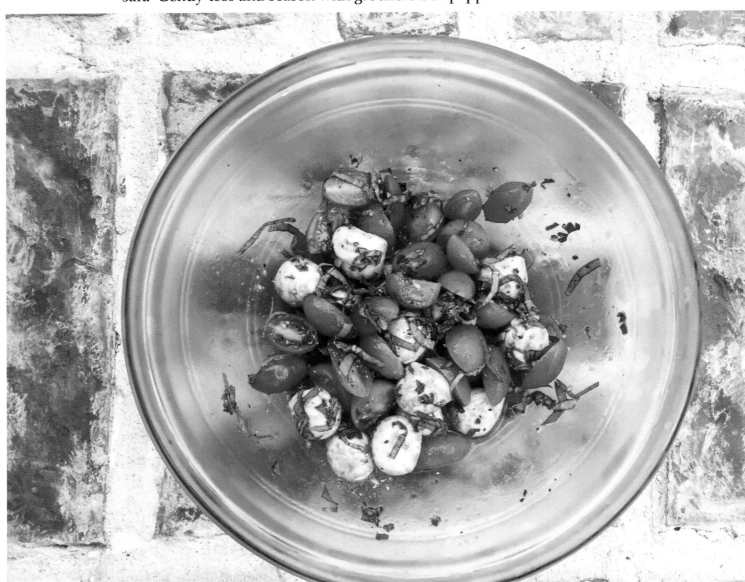

Cauliflower Fried Rice

Prep: 10 minutes
Cook: 15 minutes

1 large head of cauliflower, cleaned
1 tablespoon canola oil
2 extra large eggs
2 tablespoon canola oil
2 cloves garlic, minced
½ shallot, minced
½ cup frozen peas and carrots, thawed
½ cup frozen corn, thawed
1 teaspoon sesame oil
2 tablespoons soy sauce

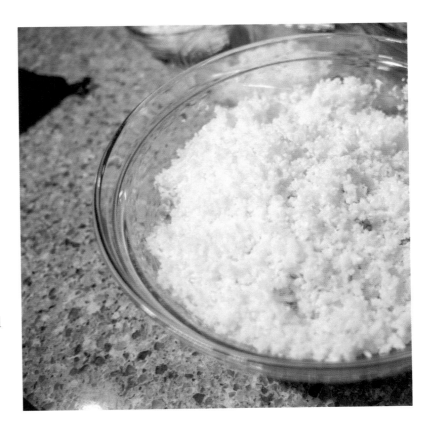

1. Chop cauliflower into 2 inch pieces, remove stems. Place cauliflower into food processor and pulse until rice/couscous like grains. If you do not have a food processor, leave the stem on and grate the cauliflower. Discard the stem once the florets are grated.

2. In a large pan or wide wok over medium high heat, add 1 tablespoon canola oil and 2 eggs. Scramble and cook for 1 minute. Remove from pan and set aside.

3. In the same pan, add 2 tablespoons canola oil, garlic and shallots. Saute for until fragrant and add cauliflower. Continue to saute for 5-7 minutes or until moisture from cauliflower is drier.

4. Add peas, carrots, corn to pan and continue to saute for 3 minutes. Add in eggs and break apart into smaller pieces while stir-frying mixture. Drizzle sesame oil and soy sauce evenly over mixture and continue to saute until combined well. Serve forth.

Summer Beef and Veggie Medley

Serves [6]
Prep: 15 minutes
Cook: 20 minutes

1 tablespoon coconut oil
1 pound grass fed ground beef (90/10)
1 tablespoon ground cumin
1 tablespoon fennel seeds
1 teaspoon coriander
Fresh cracked black pepper to taste
2 teaspoons Kosher salt
1 large onion, diced
1 bunch of kale, cleaned, shredded
1 cup cooked red beans (or black beans)
4 mini Portobello mushrooms, sliced
1 cup cherry tomatoes, diced
Grated Parmesan cheese
Sesame seeds for topping
1 bunch of fresh parsley (or cilantro) for topping
½ whole avocado, sliced (optional)

1. In a large pan over medium high heat, add coconut oil and ground beef. Sauté ground beef in coconut oil until medium doneness. Add cumin, fennel seeds, coriander, salt and pepper and continue to cook for 2 minutes.

2. Add onions and Kosher salt. Continue to sauté for 3 minutes.

3. Add in shredded kale, cooked red beans, and sliced mushrooms to pan. Cook for 10 minutes.

4. Remove from heat into serving dish. Mix diced cherry tomatoes into beef. Sprinkle parmesan cheese, top with sesame seeds and parsley or cilantro. Place sliced avocado on top and enjoy.

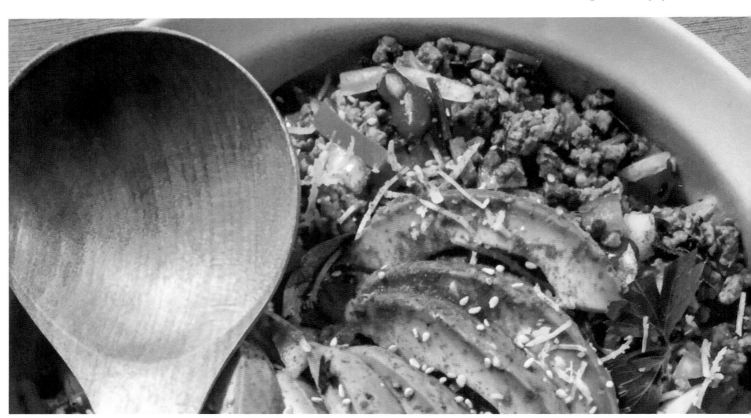

Sunset Veggie Medley

1 cup Tzatziki sauce
1 teaspoon fresh dill
2 teaspoons grated Parmesan cheese
½ teaspoon caraway seeds
½ teaspoon sesame seeds
Pinch of cinnamon
Pinch of ground cumin
Pinch of paprika
1 whole red bell pepper
1 whole yellow bell pepper
1 whole orange bell pepper
1 whole cucumber

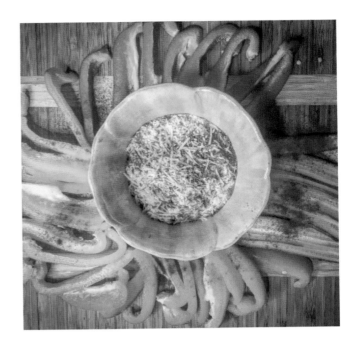

1. In a serving bowl, top Tzatziki sauce with dill, Parmesan, caraway seeds, sesame seeds, cinnamon, cumin and paprika. Set aside.

2. Remove top of bell peppers and cut out seeds and ribs. Slice into ¼ inch pieces. Cut ends off of cucumber and slice into ½ inch slices. Serve with Tzatziki sauce and enjoy cold.

Grilled Zucchini

Simple: Slice zucchini and brush with olive oil on both sides. Turn the heat on high on the grill and lay the sliced zucchini on. Sprinkle with sea salt afterward and enjoy!

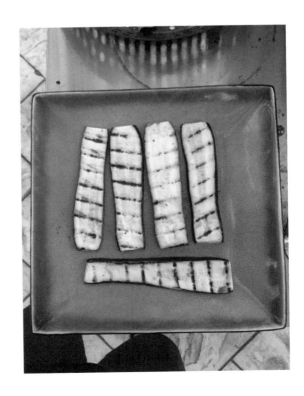

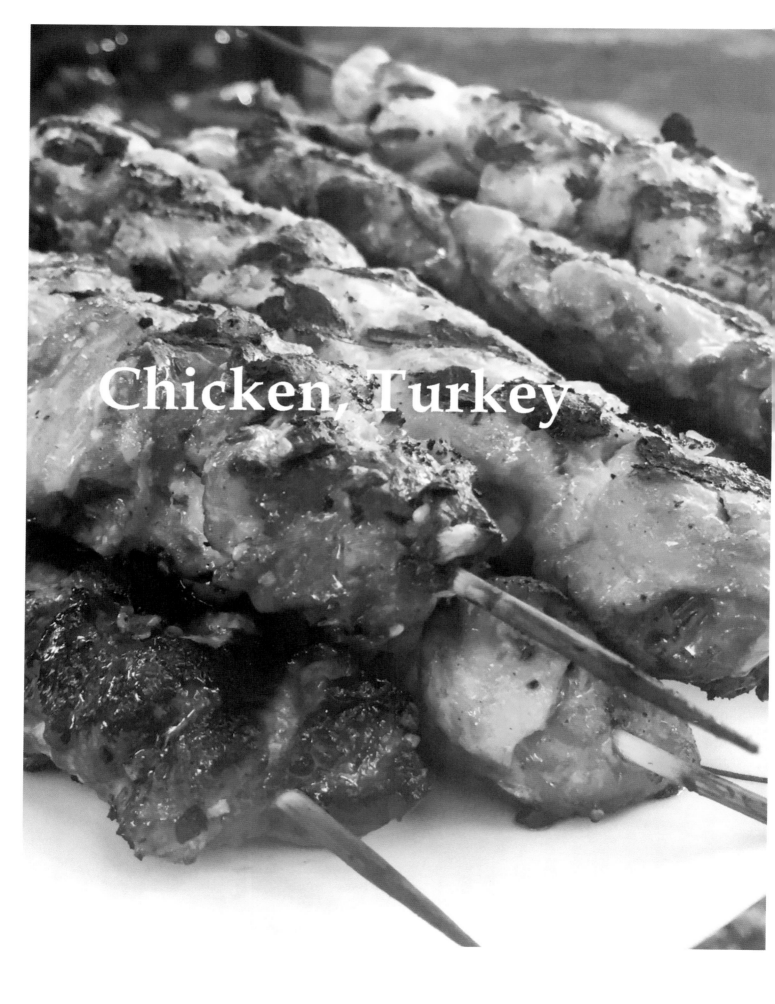

Chicken, Turkey

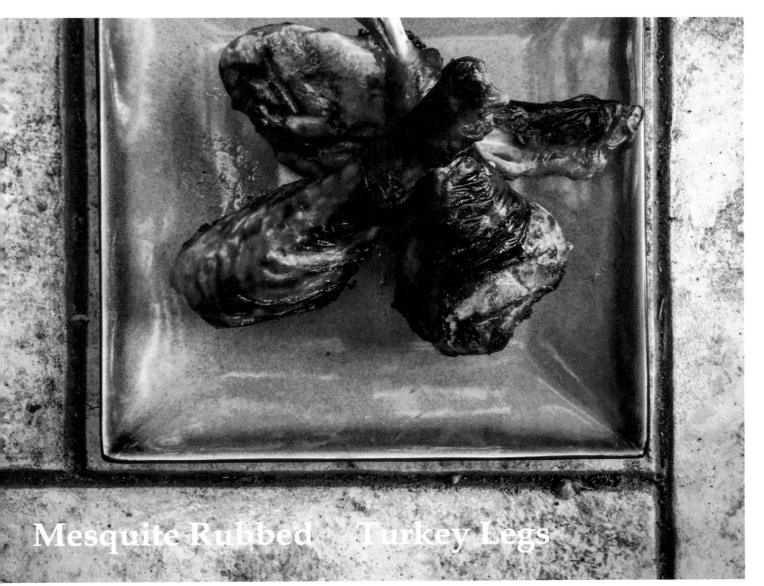

Mesquite Rubbed Turkey Legs

Serves [4]
Prep: 5 minutes
Cook: 30-40 minutes

4 whole turkey legs (skin on)
2 tablespoon mesquite seasoning

1. Coat turkey legs with seasoning.

2. Turn on the grill and heat till 400°F. Place turkey legs on the top rack of your grill and close the cover for 15 minutes. Turn the legs to the other side and cover again for 15 minutes.

3. Open cover and place turkey legs on the highest part of the grill for searing, approximately 1-2 minutes on two sides. Cook until juices run clear or internal temperature reads 170°F. Serve immediately.

Curried Chicken Soup

Serves [8]
Prep: 15 minutes
Cook 45 minutes

4 tablespoons sesame oil
½ cup chopped onions
1 tablespoon grass fed butter
2 pounds chicken (cut of any preference)
½ cup Thai Curry Paste
2 quarts chicken stock (or turkey)
Kosher salt and ground black pepper to taste
¼ cup fresh parsley, chopped

1. In a large soup pot over medium high heat, add sesame oil and coat bottom of pan. Add in onions and butter. Sauté for 2 minutes. Add in chicken pieces. Sauté until chicken has slightly browned and opaque looking (8-10 minutes depending on cut). Add in curry paste and mix well. Continue to cook for 1 minute until fragrant.

2. Pour in chicken stock and bring to a boil. Lower heat and simmer for 30 minutes.

3. Season with salt and pepper to taste. Add parsley and serve immediately.

When you share your struggles with the world, you inspire people. What is unexpected is that these people will in turn inspire you to help them.

Dr. Cheng Ruan

Lemon Chicken with Sugar Snap Peas

Serves [4]
Prep: 10 minutes
Cook: 25 minutes

1 pound boneless, skinless
chicken breasts
¼ teaspoon salt
⅛ teaspoon ground black pepper
3 tablespoons cornstarch
1 teaspoon canola oil
4 cups sugar snap peas, cleaned,
trimmed
2 teaspoons canola oil
1 (14 ounces) can reduced-sodium
chicken broth
3 cloves garlic, minced
¼ cup finely chopped fresh parsley
1 tablespoon freshly grated lemon zest
1 tablespoon lemon juice

1. Cut chicken breast into 1-by-2-inch strips and season with salt and pepper. Add cornstarch and coat chicken evenly. Set aside.

2. In a large nonstick skillet over medium-high heat, add 1 teaspoon canola oil. Add snap peas and stir-fry for 2-3 minutes, until bright green in color. Transfer out of the pan into a large container.

3. In the same pan, add 2 teaspoons canola oil to the pan until oil glistens. Add chicken and stir fry for 4-5 minutes until lightly browned. The center should be cooked through. Remove from the pan and set aside.

4. In the same pan, add broth and garlic and cook for 6 minutes or until reduced to 1 cup of sauce. Return the chicken and snap peas to the pan and turn heat down to medium. Cook for 5 minutes. Add parsley, lemon zest and lemon juice and mix to incorporate. Serve immediately.

Asian Chicken Skewers

Serves [2-4]
Prep: 1 hour 10 minutes
Cook: 10-15 minutes

4 chicken breasts (or thighs if you prefer)
3 cloves garlic, minced
1 stalk of scallion, thinly sliced
1 tablespoons fish sauce
1 teaspoon soy sauce
1 tablespoon lemon juice
    (optional: substitute with 1 tablespoon lemon grass instead of lemon juice)

1. Clean chicken and pat dry. Cut into 1 inch pieces and set aside.

2. In a large bowl, add garlic, scallion, fish sauce, soy sauce, and lemon juice and mix together. Toss chicken into bowl and coat evenly. Marinate for 1 hour in refrigerator.

3. Skewer chicken onto bamboo skewers.

4. Turn on grill to high and place chicken skewers onto hot grill. Grill each side for 4-5 minutes or until no longer pink. Serve hot.

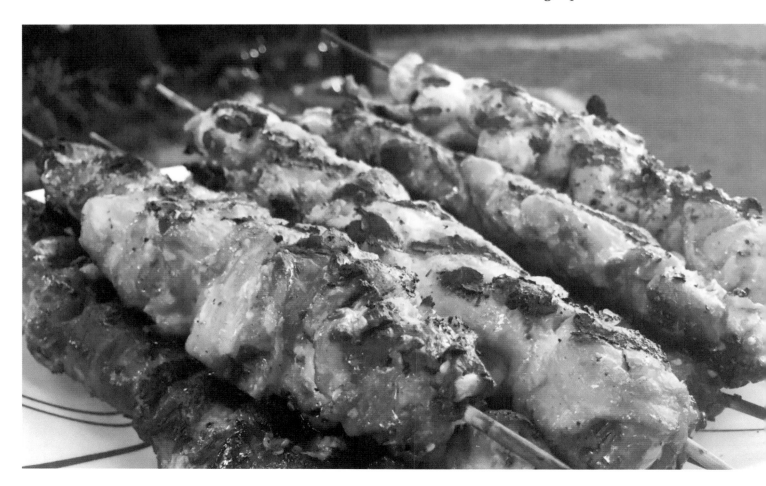

Chicken and Purple

Serves [8]
Prep: 10 minutes
Cook: 25 minutes

3 pounds chicken thighs, boneless
1 package chicken seasoning mix
1 large red onion, diced
2 tablespoons sesame oil
1 head of purple cabbage, shredded
1 teaspoon fresh thyme (chopped)
1 whole lime
2 tablespoons fish sauce
2 tablespoons sesame seeds
2 tablespoons hemp seeds
1 tablespoons ground flax seeds
Fresh cracked black pepper to taste
Fresh Parsley chopped for garnish

1. Clean and trim chicken thighs.
    Pat dry and season with chicken
    seasoning. Mix until well coated.
    Set aside.

2. Heat up grill to high heat. Grill
    chicken until fully cooked (8
    minutes per side). Cut grilled
    chicken to strips. Set aside.

3. In a large pan over medium high,
    add sesame oil and onions. Sauté
    for 5-10 minutes until
    caramelized. Add in purple
    cabbage and continue to cook
    until translucent.

4. Add fish sauce, lime juice,
    sesame seeds, hemp seeds,
    ground flax seeds. Season with
    fresh cracked black pepper.

5. Pour mixture into serving dish
    and place chopped chicken on
    top. Garnish with fresh parsley
    and serve immediately.

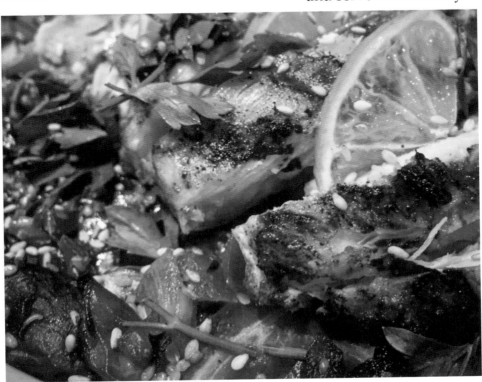

Rosemary Balsamic Chicken

Serves [4]
Prep: 10 minutes
Cook: 10 minutes
Marinate: 5 hours

4 chicken breast halves, skinless, boneless (approx. 1 pound)
1 tablespoon paprika
1 tablespoon olive oil
½ teaspoon fresh rosemary, chopped
2 cloves garlic, minced
¼ teaspoon ground black pepper
1 teaspoon olive oil
¼ cup dry red wine or water
3 tablespoons balsamic vinegar
Fresh rosemary sprigs (garnish, optional)

1. Place a piece of chicken breast between two pieces of plastic wrap and pound until ½ inch thick. Repeat until all chicken is prepped.

2. In a small bowl, combine paprika, oil, rosemary, garlic, and black pepper. Mix until paste texture. Rub entire chicken breasts with mixture.

3. In a large baking dish, coat with 1 teaspoon olive oil. Place marinated chicken in this pan, cover and refrigerate for 5 hours.

4. Preheat oven to 450°F. Evenly pour red wine over chicken breasts. Bake for 6 minutes. Turning once halfway through baking; chicken should no longer be pink and the juices should run clear.

5. Remove from oven. Immediately drizzle balsamic vinegar onto cooked chicken in the baking pan. Transfer chicken to serving plates.

6. Stir the juices in baking pan and drizzle over chicken. Garnish with rosemary sprig and serve forth.

Asian Pineapple Chicken Stir-Fry

Serves [6]
Prep: 10 minutes
Cook: 10 minutes

1 tablespoon canola oil
1 medium red onion, halved and sliced
¼ of a fresh pineapple, peeled, cored, 1 inch pieces
¾ cup zucchini, peeled, cut to 1 inch pieces
¾ cup fresh snap peas, cleaned, trimmed
3 skinless, boneless chicken breast halves, 1 inch strips
3 tablespoons stir-fry sauce (available in Asian grocery stores)

1. In a wok or large skillet over medium high heat, add 1 tablespoon canola oil. Add red onion and stir fry for 2 minutes. Add pineapple, zucchini, and snap peas and continue to stir-fry for 2 minutes. Pour into a dish and set aside.

2. In same wok or skillet, add 2 teaspoons oil to hot wok. Add chicken and stir-fry for 3 minutes or until chicken is tender and opaque. Return pineapple and vegetables to pan and continue to stir fry. Add stir-fry sauce and cook for 1 minute until everything is well coated and warmed through. Serve immediately.

The most important thing in the world is to have a WHY. If the reason is good enough, you will do it. Many people slack off because their WHY is either not strong enough, or they are not constantly reminded of their WHY.

Dr. Cheng Ruan

Chinese Honey Chicken Stir-Fry with Cashews

Serves [2]
Prep: 10 minutes
Cook: 15 minutes

1 teaspoon canola oil
¼ cup diagonally sliced carrots
¼ cup celery, cut same as carrots
2 teaspoons canola oil
8 ounces chicken breasts, skinless, boneless, cut into 1-inch pieces
¼ cup orange juice
1 teaspoon cornstarch
1 tablespoon soy sauce
1 teaspoon honey
¼ teaspoon grated fresh ginger
2 tablespoons cashews
Chopped scallions (garnish)

1. In a small bowl, whisk together orange juice and cornstarch. Add soy sauce, honey, and ginger and continue to whisk until incorporated. Set aside.

2. In a wok or large skillet over high heat, add 1 teaspoon canola oil. Add carrot and celery and stir-fry for 2 minutes. Remove from wok and set aside.

3. In same wok or skillet, add 2 teaspoons vegetable oil. Add chicken and stir fry for 4 minutes or until done. Add cooked carrots and celery back into chicken and continue to stir fry.

4. Add soy sauce mixture to wok and stir until coated. Cook over medium heat until thickened sauce thickens. Top with cashews, scallions and serve immediately.

Friend power is far stronger than self power. Having an accountability partner is vital to success.

Dr. Cheng Ruan

Stewed Louisiana Chicken Drumsticks

Serves [4]
Prep: 10 minutes
Cook: 40 minutes

1 tablespoon canola oil
8 chicken drumsticks
1 (14.5 ounce) can stewed tomatoes, no salt added,
1 cup frozen cut okra
1 tablespoon Louisiana hot sauce
¼ teaspoon salt
¼ teaspoon ground black pepper
1 teaspoon dried thyme
½ tablespoon Louisiana hot sauce

1. In a large nonstick skillet over medium-high heat, add canola oil when pan is hot. Pat chicken dry with paper towels and place into pan. Brown chicken on all sides.

2. Add stewed tomatoes, okra, 1 tablespoon hot sauce, salt and pepper. Take dried thyme and crush between the palms of your hand to until ground. Add to skillet and mix well. Bring to a boil over medium-high heat. Reduce to simmer, cover and cook for 30 minutes. Internal temperature of chicken should be 165°F or no longer pink in the center.

3. Place the chicken pieces on a serving platter. Stir the remaining hot sauce into skillet and spoon sauce over cooked chicken. Serve forth.

Low Carb Chicken Tenders

Serves [4]
Prep: 10 minutes
Cook: 30 minutes

Canola oil
2 egg whites
1 tablespoon water
¾ cup almond meal
2 tablespoons grated Parmesan cheese
¼ teaspoon garlic powder
¼ teaspoon dried parsley
¼ teaspoon ground black pepper
12 ounces chicken breast tenderloins, cut into 8 pieces
Cooking spray

1. Preheat oven to 425°F. In a baking pan, lightly coat the dish with canola oil.

2. In a small bowl, whisk together egg whites and water.

3. In a shallow dish, combine almond meal, Parmesan cheese, garlic powder, dried parsley, and black pepper. Whisk until well mixed.

4. Dip each chicken tenderloin into the egg white mixture. Next, coat with the almond meal mixture. Place breaded chicken tenders on the prepared baking pan.

5. Lightly coat breaded chicken tenders with cooking spray. Bake for 15 to 20 minutes or until crisp. Serve immediately.

Kale Caesar with Chicken and Crispy Artichokes

Serves [8]
Prep: 15 minutes
Cook: 30 minutes

Kale prep

1 bunch lacinato kale, ribs removed, coarse chop
1 tablespoon fresh lemon juice
¼ teaspoon salt

Caesar dressing:

¼ cup buttermilk
1 tablespoon extra-virgin olive oil
⅓ cup grated Pecorino Romano
1 tablespoon Worcestershire sauce
1 clove garlic, minced
½ teaspoon fresh ground black pepper
1 tablespoon fresh lemon juice

Crispy Artichokes:

Olive oil (for coating)
1/2 cup panko
1 1/2 teaspoon chopped fresh rosemary
1 tablespoon grated Pecorino Romano
1 clove garlic, minced
¼ teaspoon fresh ground black pepper
1 large egg, beaten
1 (14 ounces) can artichoke hearts, drained, halved, and patted dry

Chicken prep:

1 tablespoon olive oil
12 ounces boneless, skinless chicken breast halves
1 red onion, thinly sliced
Kosher salt and fresh ground pepper

1. Clean kale and dry well with salad spinner. In a large bowl, add kale, 1 tablespoon lemon juice and ¼ teaspoon salt. Rub mixture with kale for 1 minute until slightly wilted.

2. In a separate bowl, add buttermilk, extra virgin olive oil, Pecorino Romano, Worcestershire sauce, minced garlic, ground pepper, and lemon juice. Whisk until well combined and set aside.

3. Place a rack 6 inches from top of the oven and preheat broiler. Lightly oil 1 baking sheet. Mix panko, rosemary, Pecorino Romano, minced garlic, and 1/4 teaspoon pepper in a shallow bowl. Whisk egg and place into separate shallow bowl. Dip artichokes one at a time in egg and panko mixture. Place battered artichokes on baking sheet.

4. On a separate baking sheet, line with parchment paper. In a medium bowl, toss chicken and onion with olive oil. Season with salt and pepper. Arrange prepped chicken in a single layer on baking sheet.

5. Broil chicken and onion for 8-10 minutes, until onion is golden and tender and chicken is cooked through. Transfer to a cutting board and let chicken rest.

6. Broil artichokes, turn halfway, until golden brown and crisp, for 6 minutes.

7. Slice chicken for salad prep. Toss kale with half of dressing. Top with chicken, onion, and artichokes. Drizzle rest of dressing prior to serving.

Grilled Chicken Paillard Salad

Serves [8]
Prep: 15 minutes
Cook: 15 minutes
Marinate: 30 minutes

⅓ cup balsamic vinegar
2 tablespoons extra-virgin olive oil
2 garlic cloves, minced
1 tablespoon chopped fresh oregano
½ teaspoon salt
½ teaspoon ground black pepper
1 ½ pounds chicken cutlets
3 red bell peppers, stemmed and seeded
Kosher salt and ground black pepper
2 romaine hearts, trimmed, 1 inch pieces
Ricotta Salata or Parmesan
2 tablespoons balsamic vinegar
1 tablespoon extra-virgin olive oil

1. Combine balsamic vinegar, extra virgin olive oil, garlic, oregano, and ½ teaspoon each salt and black pepper in a small bowl. Divide marinade between 2 zip-lock backs. Place chicken in 1 bag and bell peppers in the second bag. Seal bags and coat with marinade well. Marinate at room temperature, turning bags occasionally, for 30 minutes.

2. Preheat grill to 450°F. Remove chicken and bell peppers from bags and discard marinade. Grill chicken and bell peppers, sprinkling with salt and black pepper. Cook for 4-5 minutes until peppers are soft and chicken is opaque. Transfer to a cutting board; let chicken rest for 5 minutes before slicing.

3. Place romaine lettuce into salad bowl. Slice chicken and bell peppers into strips and add to romaine lettuce. Shave ricotta salata over salad. Drizzle with vinegar and oil. Toss and serve forth.

Asian Peanut Noodles with Chicken

Serves [4]
Prep: 15 minutes
Cook: 5 minutes

1 cup cooked fettuccine noodles
2 cups chopped roasted skinless, boneless chicken breasts
2 cups thinly sliced red bell pepper
1 teaspoon dark sesame oil
2 garlic cloves, minced
1 tablespoon minced fresh ginger
⅔ cup water
⅓ cup natural-style smooth peanut butter
⅓ cup hoisin sauce
1 tablespoon seasoned rice wine vinegar
½ teaspoon Asian chili sauce
½ cup chopped fresh cilantro

1. Combine pasta, chicken and bell peppers in a large bowl.

2. In a small saucepan over medium-high heat, add sesame oil, garlic and ginger. Cook 1 minute, stirring frequently. Add water, peanut butter, hoisin sauce, rice wine vinegar and chili sauce. Whisk and continue to cook for 1 minute.

3. Pour peanut butter mixture onto pasta mixture. Toss to coat. Stir in cilantro and serve forth.

Baked Italian Chicken Breasts

Serves [4]
Prep: 10 minutes
Cook: 50 minutes

Cooking spray
1 tablespoon dried parsley
1 tablespoon dried basil
½ teaspoon salt
½ teaspoon crushed red pepper flakes
4 skinless, boneless chicken breast, halved
4 cloves garlic, thinly sliced
2 tomatoes, sliced

1. Preheat oven to 350ºF. Coat a medium sized baking dish with cooking spray.

2. In a small bowl, combine parsley, basil, salt and red pepper flakes. Stir to mix well. Coat chicken breast with mixture and place in baking dish.

3. Sprinkle evenly with garlic slices. Top with tomato slices.

4. Cover with foil and bake for 25 minutes. Remove cover, and continue baking 15 minutes or until internal temperature of chicken is 165ºF.

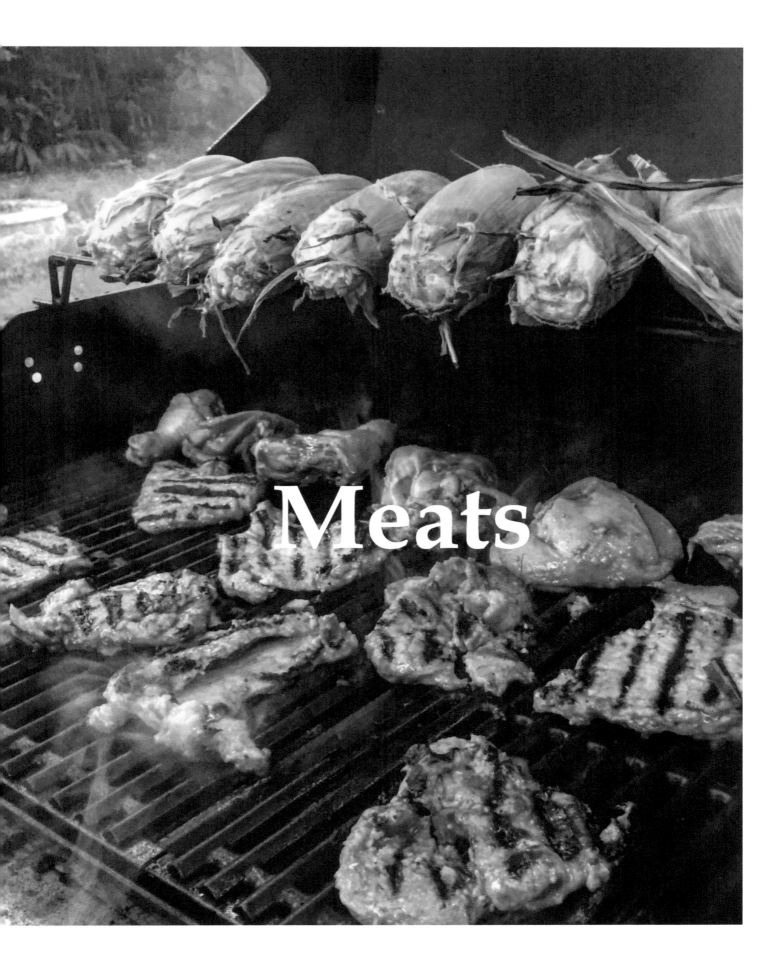

Meats

Pan Seared Sirloin Steak with Thyme and Garlic

Serves [2]
Prep: 5 minutes
Cook: 10 minutes
Rest: 10 minutes

2 (1 inch thick) sirloin steaks
Kosher salt and pepper
1 tablespoon canola oil
7 sprigs of fresh thyme
4 cloves garlic (crushed)

1. Preheat oven to 450°F. Pat steak dry with paper towels and coat both side of the steak with salt and pepper.

2. Heat large oven proof frying pan on high heat and add canola oil. Place steak into pan to sear for 2 minutes on each side. Look for a golden brown. Add thyme and crushed garlic.

3. Place frying pan into oven. Flip steak after 1 minute on each side for a rare/medium rare steak. Take out of the oven and let the meat rest for 10 minutes before cutting.

Chinese 5 Spice Pork Tenderloin

Serves [4]
Prep: 5 minutes
Cook: 15 minutes
Rest: 5 minutes

1 whole pork tenderloin (1- 1 ½ pounds)
1 ½ tablespoons Chinese Five Spice powder
1 teaspoon Kosher salt
½ teaspoon ground black pepper
1 tablespoon canola oil

1. Preheat oven to 450°F. Pat tenderloin dry and coat with spices, salt and pepper.

2. In a large oven safe pan, preferably cast iron, add oil and sear on all sides until browned, approximately 2 minutes each side.

3. Place pan into oven for 10-15 minutes. Flip the tenderloin halfway during cooking, and check the internal temp for 140°F. Let it rest for 5 minutes before slicing.

Jazzed Up Steak and Eggs

Serves [2-3]
Prep: 5 minutes
Cook: 15 minutes
Rest: 5 minutes

1 pound flank steak
Kosher salt and ground black pepper
1 tablespoon olive oil
4 roma tomatoes, halved
1 teaspoon grass fed butter
4 extra large eggs
1 tablespoon fresh oregano, chopped

1. Season flank steak with Kosher salt and black pepper on both sides. Heat a large skillet over medium high heat and add olive oil.

2. Cook steak 3-4 minutes each side and remove from skillet for medium rare. Let rest for 5 minutes to let juices redistribute before cutting.

3. Place tomatoes into skillet, cut side down for 3 minutes or until browned. Remove from pan and set aside.

4. In a nonstick pan over medium heat, add butter and crack eggs into pan for sunny side up. Cover and cook for 2-3 minutes.

5. Slice flank steak, against the grain for more tender texture. Serve forth with steak, eggs, and tomatoes. Garnish with chopped oregano.

Chinese Stir Fry Beef with Bell Peppers

Serves [2-3]
Prep: 30 minutes
Cook: 10 minutes

6oz beef loin flap meat
1 teaspoon low sodium soy sauce
1 ½ teaspoons Shaoxing cooking wine
1 teaspoon grated ginger
1 teaspoon grated garlic
½ teaspoon cane sugar
Pinch of white pepper powder
¼ teaspoon cornstarch
1 teaspoon canola oil
1 whole red bell pepper
1 whole green bell pepper
2 tablespoons canola oil (separated)
3 cloves garlic, crushed
¼ cup chicken broth
1 teaspoon hoisin sauce

1. Pat loin flap meat dry and slice against the grain into ¼ inch thick pieces. In a bowl, add beef, soy sauce, cooking wine, ginger, garlic, sugar, white pepper powder, cornstarch and canola oil. Mix well together and set aside to marinate for 30 minutes.

2. Clean bell peppers and remove inside seeds and ribs. Cut into 1 inch pieces and set aside.

3. In a large pan over medium high heat, add 1 tablespoon canola oil. Place beef into heated pan and sauté for 2-3 minutes. Set aside.

4. In same pan, add remaining tablespoon canola oil and garlic. Add in bell peppers and sauté for 1 minute. Pour in chicken broth, lower heat to medium and cover pan for 2 minutes.

5. Open cover and continue to sauté until liquid is gone from the pan. Return beef into pan and add hoisin sauce. Sauté for 1 minute and serve immediately.

Grilled Herb Lamb Chops

Serves [3-4]
Prep: 6 hours
Cook: 10 minutes

¼ cup olive oil
½ cup fresh parsley
½ cup fresh oregano
8 garlic cloves, chopped
1 teaspoon Kosher salt
½ teaspoon fresh ground black pepper
Juice of 2 lemons
6 (1 inch thick) lamb chops

1. In a large bowl or baking dish, mix olive oil, parsley, oregano, garlic, salt, black pepper and lemon juice until well incorporated. Pat lamb chop dry and place into marinade. Coat all sides of lamb chop with marinade and place in fridge for 6 hours. Turn lamb chops halfway in marinade to ensure even marination.

2. Turn on grill and place lamb chops on hottest part of grill for 3 minutes. Drizzle remaining marinade on top of each chop. Flip and cook for 3 minutes. Remove from heat and let rest for 10 minutes before serving.

Stress is the number 1 killer in the world. Stress can create bad eating, sleeping, and other bad habits which can lead to many chronic diseases, including Type 2 diabetes.

Dr. Cheng Ruan

Low Carb Meatballs

Serves [8]
Prep: 45 minutes
Cook: 10 minutes

1 packet unflavored gelatin
½ cup chicken stock
1 medium onion, minced
8 cloves garlic, finely minced
½ cup fresh parsley, chopped
¾ cup grated Parmigiano-Reggiano
½ cup almond flour
3 eggs
1 teaspoon Kosher salt
½ teaspoon ground black pepper
¼ teaspoon garlic powder
1 teaspoon dried oregano
1 teaspoon ground fennel seeds
½ cup warm water
1 pound grass fed ground beef
1 pound organic ground pork

1. In a small bowl, add gelatin to chicken stock and let stand for 5 minutes. Microwave for 2 minutes and stir until gelatin is dissolved. Place in refrigerator for 30 minutes until gelatin has set.

2. Preheat oven to 350°F. In a large mixing bowl, add onion, garlic, parsley, Parmigiano-Reggiano, almond flour, eggs, salt, pepper, garlic powder, oregano, fennel seeds and warm water. Mix until incorporated.

3. Finely mince gelatin and add into bowl, stir until well distributed.

4. Add beef and pork to bowl and mix until all ingredients are well incorporated.

5. Roll meat mixture into 2 inch balls and place onto lined baking sheet. Bake for 20-30 minutes.

Note: Serve with tomato sauce and freshly chopped parsley. If you want to simmer the meatballs in tomato sauce, preheat broiler and place meatballs to broil for 7-10 minutes or until browned. Then add meatballs into pot of simmering tomato sauce for 10-20 minutes. Serve with freshly grated Parmigiano-Reggiano and fresh chopped parsley.

Shepard's Pie with Cauliflower Mash

Serves [8]
Prep: 20 minutes
Cook: 1 hour

1 head of cauliflower, cleaned, cut into pieces
4 tablespoons grass fed butter
2 tablespoons sour cream
½ teaspoon garlic powder
Kosher salt and pepper to taste
2 tablespoons olive oil
1 whole red onion, diced
2 cloves garlic, minced
1 pound grass fed ground beef (80/20)
1 (14 ounces) canned chopped tomatoes
¼ cup beef stock
1 cup carrots, small dice
½ cup fresh chopped parsley
¾ cup shredded Cheddar cheese

1. In a large saucepan over medium high heat, boil cauliflower for 10-15 minutes until soft. Drain cauliflower and place in a blender or use a handheld blender in pot after water is drained. Add butter, sour cream, garlic powder, salt and pepper and puree until smooth. If it's too watery, heat on stove for an additional 1-2 minutes. Set aside.

2. In a large pan over medium heat, add olive oil, red onion and minced garlic. Cook for 1-2 minutes, moving mixture around to ensure it doesn't burn.

3. Add ground beef to pan and cook until browned, breaking apart meat with a spatula during browning process.

4. Add chopped tomatoes, beef stock and carrots. Mix for 1 minute and turn down heat to simmer uncovered for 10 minutes until most of the liquid is gone from the pan. Add in fresh chopped parsley and mix to incorporate. Remove from heat for assembly.

5. Preheat oven to 400°F. In a greased casserole dish, pour meat mixture and spread to an even layer. Next spread cauliflower puree as second layer. Sprinkle cheese and bake for 20-25 minutes until cheese is browned. Serve immediately, garnish with more chopped parsley if desired.

Pernil (Cuban Roasted Pork Shoulder)

Serves [10-12]
Prep: 12 hours (overnight)
Cook: 10 minutes

8 pound pork shoulder, picnic cut, bone-in
10 cloves garlic, minced
3 tablespoons olive oil
1 teaspoon oregano
1 teaspoon Kosher salt
½ teaspoon cracked black pepper
2 teaspoon white vinegar
1 teaspoon ancho chili powder
Kosher salt

1. In a medium bowl, combine garlic, olive oil, oregano, salt, cracked black pepper, white vinegar, and chili powder. Mix well until you form a paste. Set aside.

2. Wash pork shoulder and pat the meat dry. Place whole shoulder on cutting board skin side up and with a sharp knife, separate fat from meat in one layer leaving 1 inch uncut to keep the fat flap and meat still connected with each other. Peel back fat and poke deep slits into meat (1 -1 ½ inch deep) all over pork shoulder. Rub seasoning paste all over meat and make sure it gets into slits. Return fat piece back to cover meat and season top with Kosher salt. Cover pork should with plastic wrap and refrigerate overnight.

3. Preheat oven to 400°F. Take out pork shoulder 45 minutes - 1 hour before roasting and let sit at room temperature. Place pork shoulder in deep roasting pan (at least 2 inch deep to catch fat and juices) and roast for 1 hour, uncovered. Turn down temp to 300°F and continue to roast for 4 hours, do not baste or turn over meat to ensure crispy crust.

4. Remove pork shoulder from oven and let rest 30 minutes. Cut off crispy fat cap from meat completely before carving. Cut into smaller pieces and serve on top of carved mea

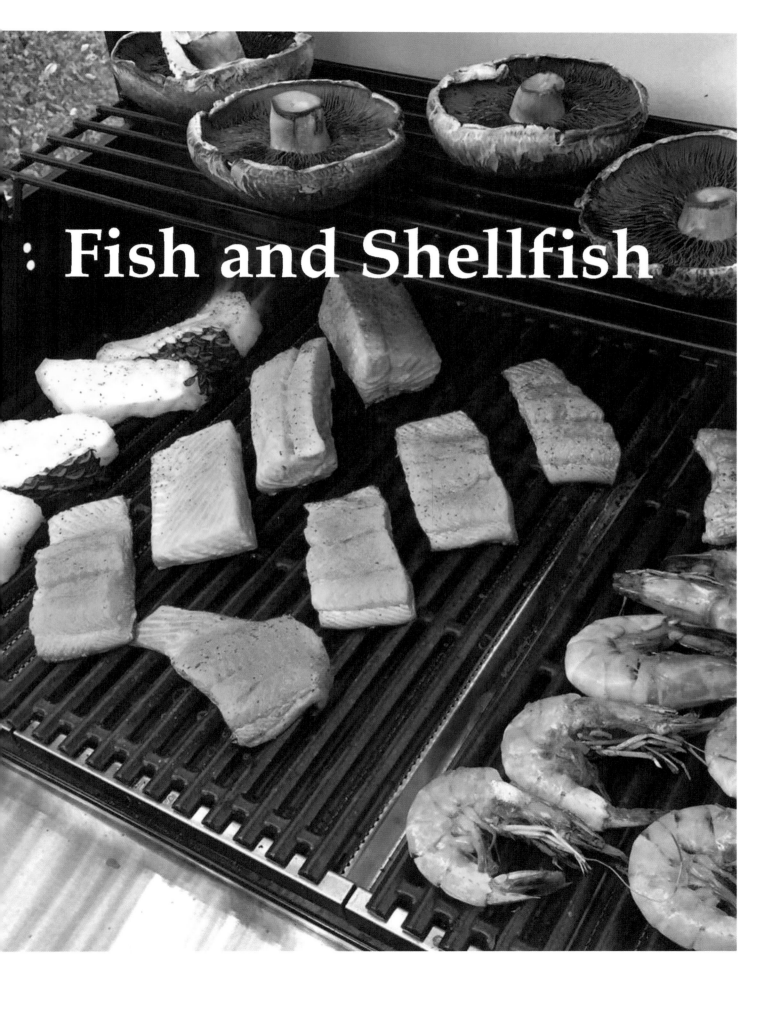

: Fish and Shellfish

Octopus Salad

Serves [8]
Prep: 10 minutes
Cook: 2 hours

1 whole octopus (4-5 pounds)
½ cup olive oil
1 cup diced celery
Juice of 4 lemons
1 clove garlic, minced
½ cup red onion, thinly sliced
1 tablespoon fresh parsley, chopped
¼ cup extra virgin olive oil
2 tablespoons red wine vinegar
Kosher salt and black pepper to taste

1. In a large stock pot, place octopus, oil and salt and boil for about 1 hour 30 minutes to 2 hours. Octopus should be tender when you stick a fork in the thickest part. Drain, discard head and clean.

2. Slice tentacles and add to a bowl. Add celery, lemon juice, garlic, onion, parsley and extra virgin olive oil. Season with Kosher salt and pepper and toss well.

3. Serve at room temperature.

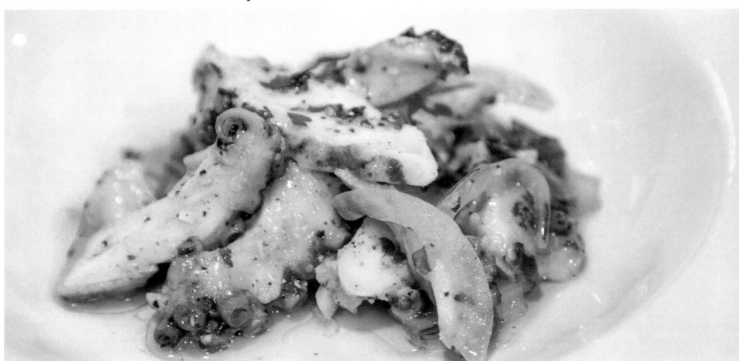

Grilled Salmon Collar

Serves [6]
Prep: 5 minutes
Cook: 10 minutes

6 wild Alaskan salmon collars
2 teaspoons sea salt
2 teaspoons white pepper powder
1 whole lemon

1. Heat up grill to high. Wash salmon collars and pat dry. Season with salt and pepper on all sides.

2. Place collar skin side down on heated grill. Cook for 5 minutes. Flip and cook for 5 minutes on other side. Cut lemon in half and squeeze juice over collar before serving.

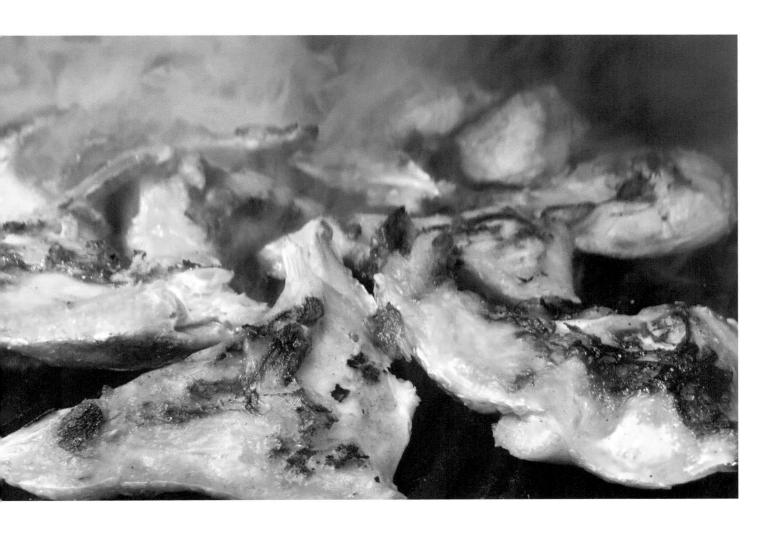

Mediterranean Grilled Octopus

Serves [4]
Prep: 5 minutes
Cook: 1 hour

1 large octopus (3 pounds)
1 cup of white wine
1 bay leaf
1 tablespoon dried thyme
1 tablespoon sea salt
2 tablespoons peppercorn
1 whole lemon
1 tablespoon olive oil
½ whole lemon
Fresh cracked black pepper to taste

1. Wash and clean octopus. In a large stock pot, combine octopus, white wine, bay leaf, dried thyme, sea salt, and peppercorns to pot. Cut lemon in half and squeeze juice of 1 lemon into pot. Pour filtered water over octopus until covering entire octopus.

2. Bring to a boil and simmer for 40 minutes. Take out octopus and discard contents.

3. Heat grill on high, and grill octopus on all sides until nice smoky char on outside.

4. Remove from grill and slice into individual tentacle pieces. Drizzle with olive oil. Squeeze lemon juice over octopus. Season with freshly cracked black pepper and serve forth.

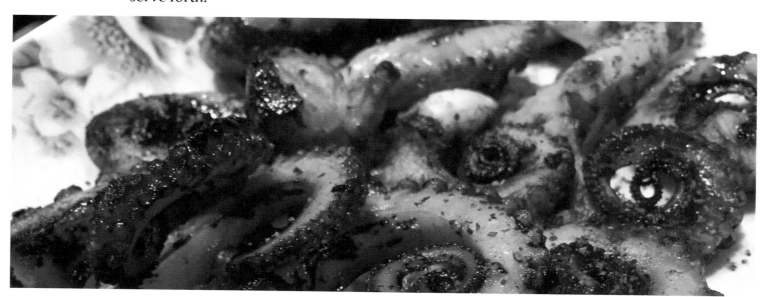

Sesame Ahi Tuna on Purple

Serve [4]
Prep: 10 minutes
Cook: 10 minutes

2 (3 ounces) Ahi tuna steaks (preferably sashimi grade)
1 teaspoon sea salt
¼ teaspoon ground black pepper
1 tablespoon ground cumin
1 teaspoon paprika
¼ cup sesame seeds (for crust)
1 tablespoon sesame oil
½ head of purple cabbage, shredded
½ cup greek yogurt (plain, full fat)
1 tablespoon fresh dill
10 whole cherry tomatoes
1 whole lime
Pinch of fennel seeds
Sesame seeds (garnish)

1. Pat tuna steaks dry and season all sides with sea salt, pepper, cumin, and paprika. Pour sesame seeds onto separate dish and roll seasoned tuna onto sesame seeds. Pat down to make sure tuna steaks are encrusted with sesame seeds. Set aside.

2. In a large pan over high heat, add sesame oil and swirl to coat pan. Sear tuna on each side until desired doneness. For sashimi grade ahi, sear for 1-2 minutes on each side for rare. Remove from pan and let sit for 2 minutes.

3. In a large bowl, add purple cabbage, dill, and yogurt. Mix well and add cherry tomatoes. Place into serving dish.

4. Slice tuna and place on top of cabbage mixture. Cut lime in half and squeeze juice over dish. Sprinkle with fennel seeds and sesame seeds and serve immediately.

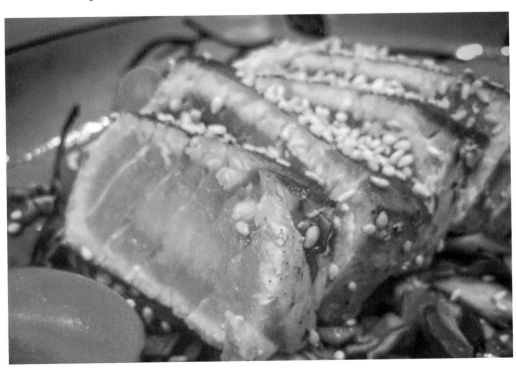

Seared Scallops

Serve [1-2]
Prep: 5 minutes
Cook: 5 minutes

6 large whole scallops
Pinch of sea salt
¼ teaspoon ground black pepper
⅛ teaspoon paprika
Pinch of ground cumin
1 tablespoon coconut oil
Grated Parmesan cheese
1 lime wedge for squeezing

1. Pat scallops dry. Season with salt, pepper, paprika and cumin. Set aside.

2. In a large nonstick pan over high heat, add coconut oil and swirl to coat bottom. Sear scallops for 2 minutes on each side for medium rare.

3. Sprinkle with grated parmesan and squeeze lime juice over scallops. Serve hot.

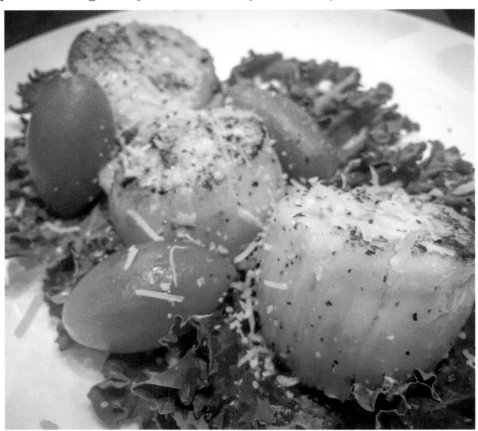

Shrimp with Healthy Plant Mix

Serve [6]
Prep: 10 minutes
Cook: 10 minutes

2 tablespoons sesame oil
½ head purple cabbage, shredded
1 whole carrot, thinly sliced
½ head cauliflower
⅓ cup pumpkin seeds
½ cup shredded kelp/seaweed
1 teaspoon sea salt
2 pounds cooked shrimp, peeled and deveined
Ground black pepper to taste
1 whole lime

1. In a large skillet over high heat, add sesame oil and swirl to coat pan. Add cabbage, carrots, cauliflower, pumpkin seeds and kelp. Season with sea salt and cook for 8 minutes.

2. Toss in shrimp into same pan and season with ground black pepper to taste.

3. Remove from heat and place into serving dish. Cut lime in half and squeeze lime juices over dish before serving.

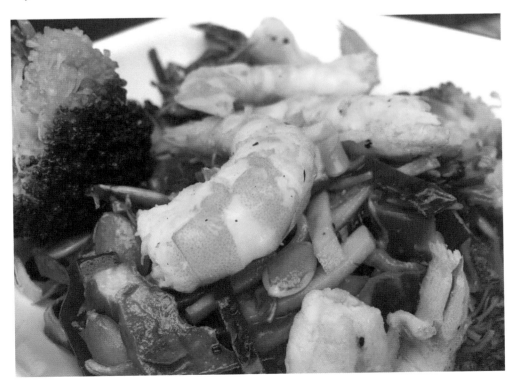

Shrimp Taco in Chickpea Tortilla

Serve [4]
Prep: 10 minutes
Cook: 10 minutes

1 tablespoon sesame oil
12 whole shrimps, peeled and deveined
1 teaspoon ground cumin
1 teaspoon paprika
Kosher salt and ground black pepper to taste
1 batch of chickpea tortillas (see "Chickpea Tortillas")
1 cup shredded cabbage
½ cup chopped tomatoes
¼ cup sliced red bell peppers
1 whole avocado, sliced
½ cup fresh parsley, chopped

1. In a large pan over high heat, add sesame oil and add shrimp, cumin and paprika. Sauté for 5 minutes and season with salt and pepper to taste. Remove from heat and set aside to cool for 10 minutes.

2. For assembly, top each tortilla piece with cabbage, chopped tomatoes, red bell peppers, avocado slices, cooked shrimp and chopped parsley. Serve wrapped.

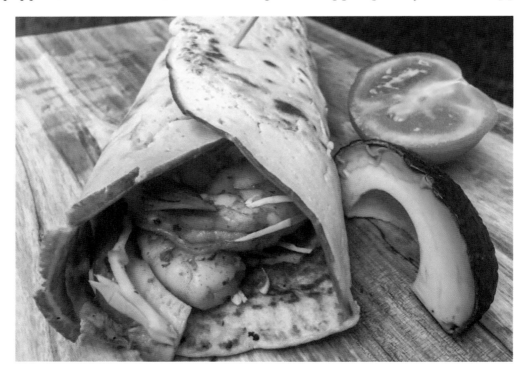

Baked Salmon with Mustard Dill Sauce

Serves [4]
Prep: 30 minutes
Cook: 10 minutes

1 cup sour cream
3 tablespoons Dijon mustard 1 whole
shallot, minced
2 cloves garlic, minced
½ cup fresh dill, chopped
¼ cup fresh parsley, chopped
Kosher salt and fresh cracked black
pepper to taste
1½ pounds salmon fillets, skin on
4 lemon wedges

1. In a medium bowl, whisk sour cream, mustard, shallot, garlic, dill, and parsley together. Season with salt and pepper to taste.

2. Preheat oven to 400°F. Pat salmon dry and cut into 4 equal pieces. Season each salmon fillet with Kosher salt and black pepper. On a lined baking sheet, place each fillet skin side down and top each with mustard sauce. Bake for 15-20 minutes. Serve with lemon wedge.

Almond Parmesan Crusted Cod

Serves [4]
Prep: 10 minutes
Cook: 12-15 minutes

1 tablespoon olive oil
½ cup almond meal
¼ cup grated Parmigiano-Reggiano
¼ cup fresh parsley, chopped
½ teaspoon garlic powder
¼ teaspoon ground black pepper
4 (6 ounce) fillets of fresh cod
4 tablespoons grass fed butter
Sea salt and fresh ground black pepper
4 lemon wedges

1. In a bowl, combine olive oil, almond meal, Parmigiano-Reggiano, parsley, garlic powder and ground black pepper. Mix well and set aside.

2. Preheat oven to 450°F. Clean cod and pat dry. Rub 1 tablespoon of grass fed butter on each fillet. Season with sea salt and fresh ground pepper on both sides. Top each fillet with almond meal mixture and pat down to adhere crust.

3. On a lined baking sheet, place prepared fillets and cook for 10-12 minutes, or until cod flakes easily with a fork. Remove and serve with lemon wedges immediately

Pan Seared Red Snapper with Lime Cilantro Sauce

Serves [4]
Prep: 10 minutes
Cook: 10 minutes

1 tablespoon olive oil
4 (6 ounce) fillets red snapper, skin on
Kosher salt and ground black pepper
2 tablespoons grass fed butter
1 tablespoon chopped shallots
3 tablespoons chopped cilantro
2 cloves garlic, minced
Juice of 1 lime
Lime zest from 1 lime
4 lime wedges

1. In a large nonstick pan over medium heat, add olive oil. Season fillets with Kosher salt and ground black pepper and place skin side down into pan. Sear for 3-4 minutes on each side. Remove from heat and place on serving dish

2. In same pan, add butter, shallots, cilantro, garlic, lime juice and lime zest. Stir for 1 minute and pour over snapper. Pour over snapper and serve with lime wedges.

Grilled Whole Trout

Serves [2-3]
Prep: 12 hours (overnight)
Cook: 10 minutes

2 (1 pound) trouts, with head and tail, gutted
Olive oil
Sea salt and freshly ground black pepper
1 lemon, thinly sliced
1 whole onion, thinly sliced
2 cloves garlic, minced
1 bunch parsley, leaves only
6 sprigs fresh thyme
Lemon wedges

1. Preheat grill to high. Rinse trouts with cold water and pat dry. Slash 6-8 slits on each side of trout. Rub whole trout generously with olive oil. Sprinkle salt and pepper inside fish cavity and outside. Divide lemon, onion, garlic, parsley and thyme in half. Stuff each cavity with these ingredients.

2. Place trout onto hot grill and cook for 6-7 minutes. Carefully flip fish to other side using 2 spatulas and continue to cook for 6-7 minutes. Serve with lemon wedges.

Steamed Fresh Tilapia with Scallions and Ginger

Serves [2]
Prep: 10 minutes
Cook: 15 minutes

1 (1½ pounds) fresh whole tilapia, head and tail intact
1 stalk scallion, julienned
4 slices ginger
2 tablespoons canola oil
1½ tablespoons seasoned soy sauce for seafood
    (available in Asian grocery stores)

1. Rinse fish in cold water and pat dry with paper towels. Place onto heatproof dish and set aside.

2. In a large pot or wok, set a steamer on the bottom and fill the pot with water (make sure water is not higher than steamer). Bring water to a boil.

3. Once boiling, set plate onto steamer and cover. Cook for 10-12 minutes or until flesh can be flaked off. Remove from heat and pour out any excess liquid on theplate during steaming process.

4. Julienne ginger pieces and set together with scallions. In a small pan over medium high heat, add canola oil to heated pan. Combine scallion and ginger and sauté for 1 minute. Remove from heat and pour in soy sauce. Stir well to combine.

5. Pour sauce over fish and serve immediately.

Most people are emotional eaters. It's how you handle those emotions that dictate success in health.

Dr. Cheng Ruan

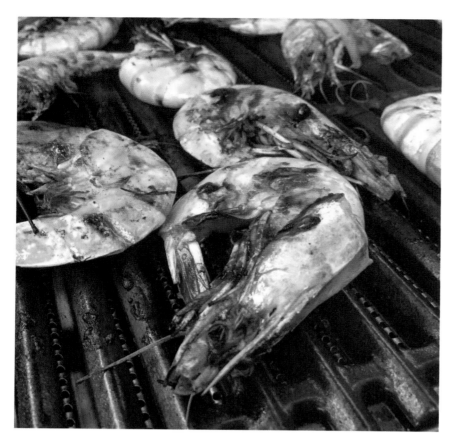

Grilled Shrimp

Seafood and more seafood

*Who says the grill is only for meat?
Pictured here is Sockeye salmon,
gulf coast shrimp, chilean sea bass,
and portobello mushrooms all
getting toasty together.*

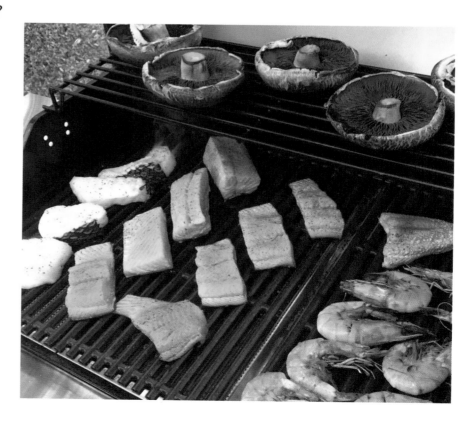

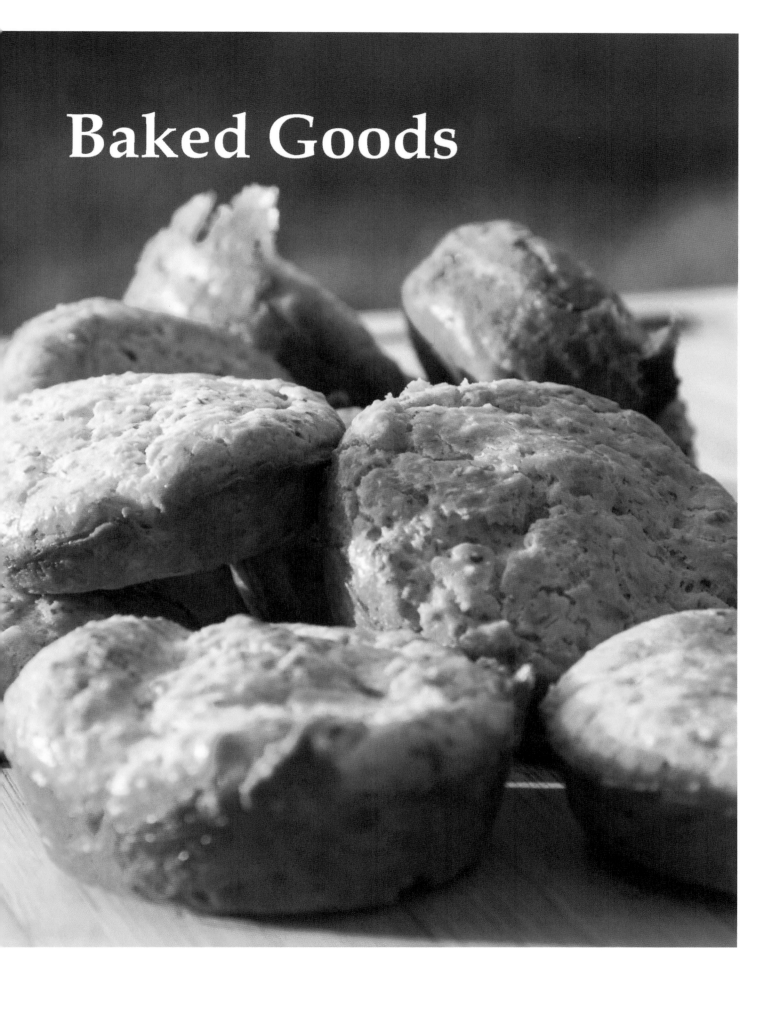

Baked Goods

Chickpea Tortillas

Serves: [4 pieces]
Prep: 10 minutes
Cook: 20 minutes

2 tablespoons ground flaxseed
2 tablespoons warm water
1 cup chickpea flour
⅔ cup water
⅛ teaspoon salt
⅛ teaspoon cumin
Canola oil

1. Combine flax meal and warm water in a large bowl. Let it rest for 5 minutes to thicken.

2. Add chickpea flour, water, salt and cumin and whisk till smooth. Look for the thickness of pancake batter.

3. In a nonstick frying pan over medium heat, add 1 teaspoon canola oil and swirl to coat the pan. Pour ½ cup of batter into the pan, swirl until the batter is even. Cook for 3 minutes or until you see the edges start to dry out. Flip and cook for another 1 minute and remove from pan. Use a clean cloth to cover cooked tortilla. Repeat until all the batter is finished.

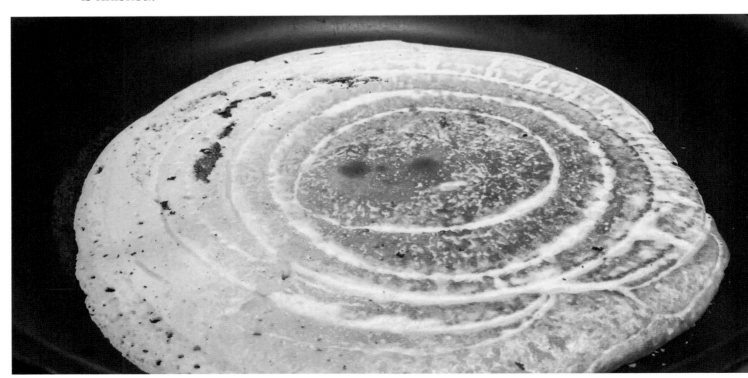

Cauliflower Pizza Crust

Prep: 10 minutes
Cook: 20-30 minutes

1 head of cauliflower
1 large egg
¾ cup shredded mozzarella and Parmesan blend
1 tablespoon Italian seasoning
¼ teaspoon Kosher salt
¼ teaspoon ground black pepper

1. Clean cauliflower and remove stem. Break into florets and rice cauliflower in a food processor.

2. Pour riced cauliflower into a heatproof bowl and microwave on high for 6 minutes, or until cooked.

3. Remove cauliflower and place into cheesecloth. Squeeze out excess moisture. Work in batches if cannot be done all at once.

4. In a large bowl, add cauliflower, egg, mozzarella and Parmesan blend, Italian seasoning, salt and pepper. Mix together very well.

5. Preheat oven to 450°F. On a lined baking sheet, pour mixture into pan and press to an even layer (approximately ½ inch thick). Bake for 20 minutes until lightly golden brown.

Note: Optional: top with tomato sauce, fresh mozzarella and salami and continue to bake for 10 minutes.

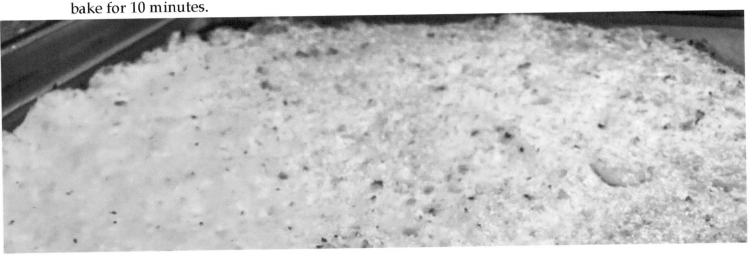

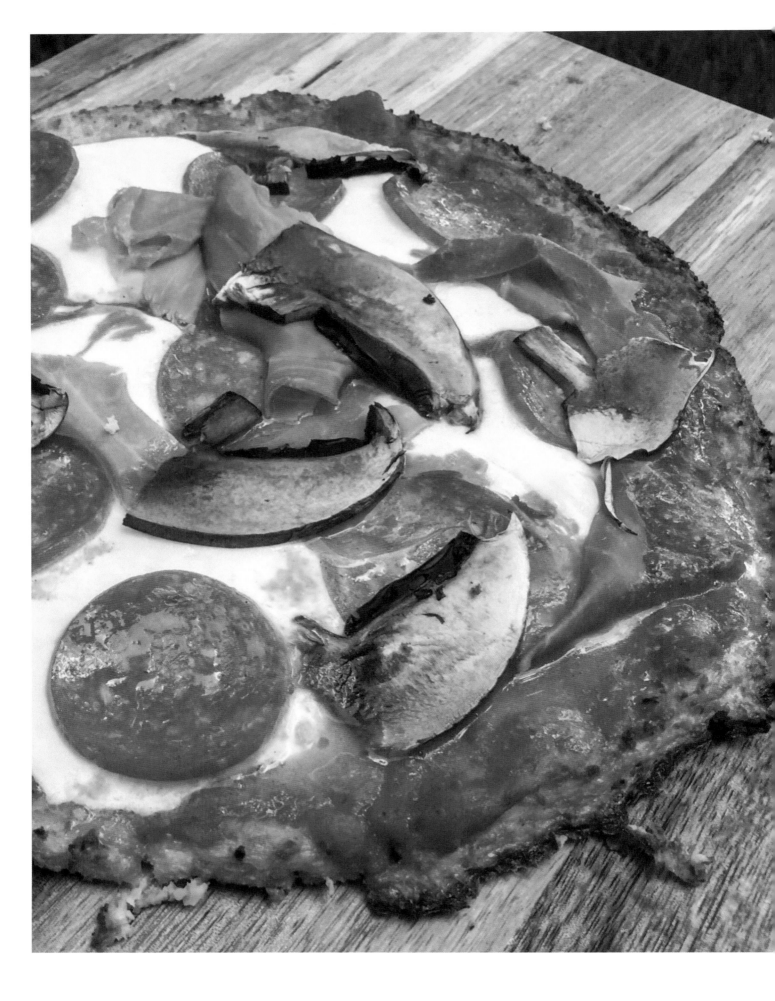

Almond Flour Cheddar Biscuits (Low Carb)

Yield: 6 biscuits
Prep: 10 minutes
Cook: 15-20 minutes

⅓ cup almond flour
1 teaspoon garlic powder
¼ teaspoon baking powder
⅛ teaspoon Kosher salt
⅛ teaspoon ground black pepper
3 large eggs
6 ounces shredded sharp cheddar cheese
⅓ cup grass fed butter

1. Preheat oven to 400°F. In a large bowl, combine almond flour, baking powder, garlic powder, salt and pepper. Mix together.

2. In a separate bowl, beat together eggs and butter until consistency is smooth. Fold into almond flour mixture, making sure there are no lumps.

3. Fold in cheddar cheese into mixture.

4. In a greased cupcake pan, spoon mixture into each. Bake for 15 minutes or until golden brown. Remove from heat and let sit for 10 minutes before serving.

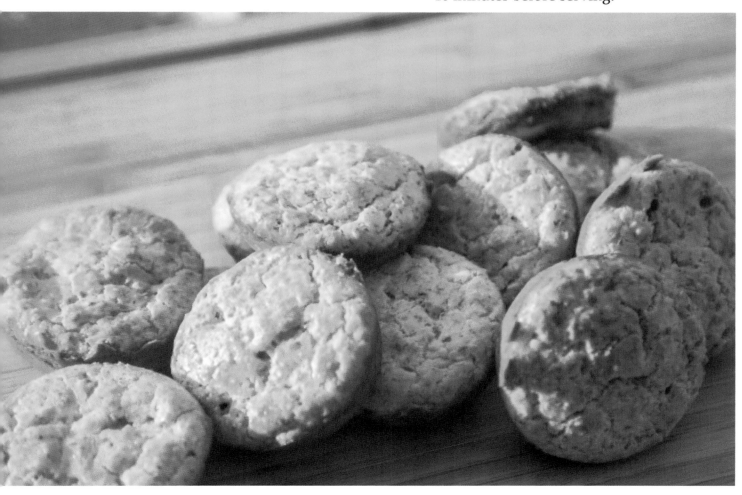

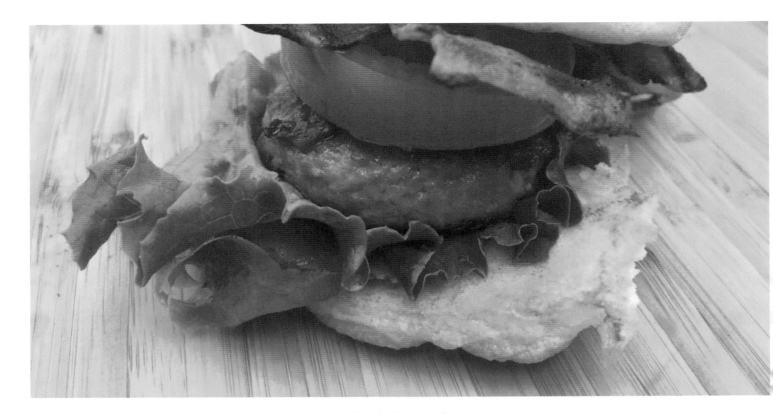

Oopsie Bread (The Ultra Low Carb Substitute)

Serves [3]
Prep: 15 minutes
Cook: 25 minutes

3 extra large egg whites
4 ounces cream cheese
1 teaspoon of table salt
½ tablespoon psyllium husk powder
½ teaspoon baking powder

1. Preheat oven to 350°F. Separate egg whites from yolks. Place into 2 separate bowls.

2. In the bowl with egg whites, add salt and whip together until stiff peaks. The texture of the mixture should be stiff enough that it doesn't move when you turn the bowl over. Set aside.

3. In the second bowl containing the egg yolks, add cream cheese and psyllium husk powder. Mix well. Fold egg whites into egg yolk mixture until well combined.

4. On a lined baking sheet, drop 6 spoonfuls of batter, evenly spaced, onto tray. Bake for 20 minutes. Cool for 5 minutes before serving.

Lemon Almond Pound Cake

Serves [8-10]
Prep: 30 minutes
Cook: 10 minutes

1½ cups almond flour (super fine)
3 tablespoons coconut flour
1 teaspoon baking soda
¼ teaspoon salt
Zest of 3 organic lemons
3 large eggs
¼ cup coconut milk
¼ cup honey
Juice of 3 organic lemons
2 teaspoons vanilla extract
2 tablespoons coconut cream
2 tablespoons coconut oil

1. Preheat oven to 350°F. In a large mixing bowl, sift together almond flour, coconut flour, baking soda, and salt. Add lemon zest and whisk to combine.

2. In a separate bowl, whisk eggs together with coconut milk, honey, lemon juice, vanilla extract, coconut cream and coconut oil. Slowly stir into flour mixture until well combined.

3. Grease loaf pan with coconut oil and line with parchment paper. Pour batter in and bake for 40 minutes or when toothpick comes out clean when inserted. Remove from oven and cool for 10 minutes before slicing.

Low Carb Chocolate Bundt Cake

Serves [12]
Prep: 15 minutes
Cook: 1 hour

2¼ cups almond flour (super fine)
¾ cup cocoa powder
1 tablespoon instant espresso powder
2 teaspoon baking soda
½ teaspoon baking powder
¼ teaspoon salt
½ cup grass fed butter, softened
⅓ cup raw honey
2 large eggs, whisked
2 teaspoons vanilla extract
½ cup coconut milk

1. Preheat oven to 325°F. Grease large bundt pan with butter and set aside. In a large bowl, sift together almond flour, cocoa powder, espresso powder, baking powder, baking soda and salt.

3. In a separate large bowl, combine butter, honey, eggs, vanilla extract and coconut milk. Whisk together until well combined. Stir in half of almond flour mixture into wet ingredient until well mixed. Stir in last half into batter, making sure there are no lumps.

2. Pour batter into greased pan and bake for 40 minutes or when toothpick comes out clean when inserted. Cool for 10-15 minutes before serving.

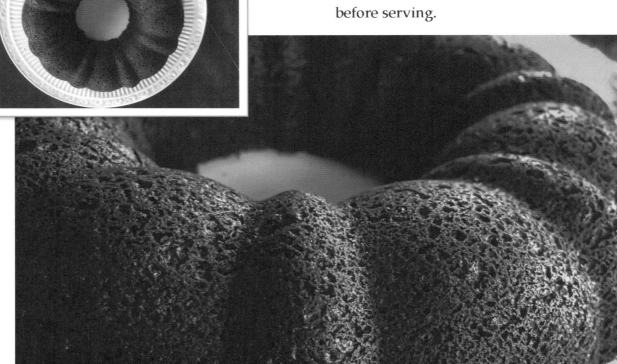

Low Carb Bread

Serves [6]
Prep: 15 minutes
Cook: 1 hour

1½ cup blanched almond flour
5 tablespoons psyllium husk powder
2 teaspoons baking powder
1 teaspoon sea salt
2 tablespoons apple cider vinegar
3 eggs whites
1 cup boiling water

1. Preheat oven to 350°F. In a large mixing bowl, sift together almond flour, psyllium husk powder, baking powder and sea salt. Whisk until well combined.

2. Add apple cider vinegar and egg whites. Mix until a doughy consistency. Pour in boiling water and continue to mix until a dough comes together.

3. Divide dough into 6 pieces and shape into mini loaves. On a greased baking sheet, place loaves onto pan and bake for 55-60 minutes. Store bread in refrigerator or freezer if not consuming immediately.

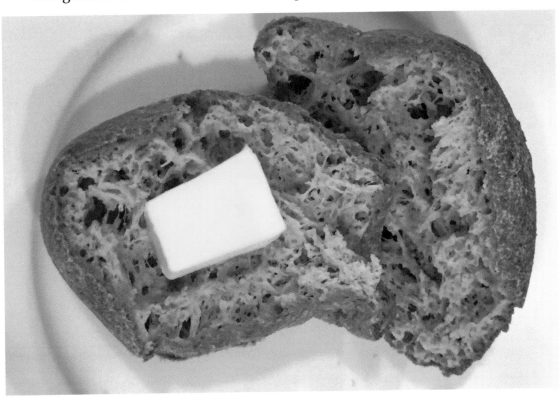

Zucchini Noodles with Creamy Avocado Pesto

Serve [6]
Prep: 10 minutes
Cook: 5 minutes

2 ripe avocados, pitted
1 tablespoon dried basil
1 clove of garlic
¼ cup pine nuts
2 tablespoon lemon juice
1 teaspoon sea salt
3 tablespoons olive oil
3 tablespoons sesame oil
4 large zucchini, spiralized
Fresh ground black pepper to taste

1. In a food processor or blender, combine avocado, basil, garlic, pine nuts, lemon juice and salt and puree until smooth. Slowly add in olive oil into food processor/blender until mixture becomes creamy. Set aside.

2. In a large pan over high heat, add sesame oil and sauté zucchini for 2 minutes.

3. Place into serving bowls and toss with sauce. Season with fresh ground black pepper to taste and serve immediately.

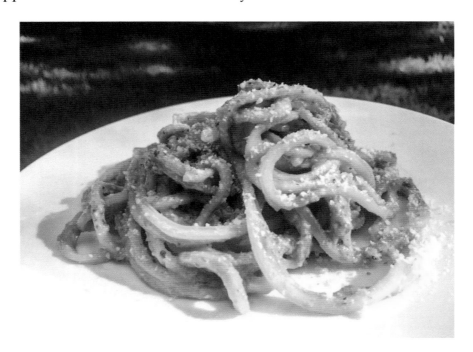

The secret to change is
to focus all of your energy,
not on fighting the old,
but on building the new.

Closing Sentiments

Thank you for putting your time and effort into reading this! I am always happy when a patient of mine walks into my office with a big smile after following this plan and gives me a hug or a high five for meeting their goals. I hope this helps you reach your goals as well! It gives me no greater pleasure than to tell my patients they no longer need their insulin or their other medications. I truly believe using food as medicine is the key to ultimate health, fitness, and happiness!

A lot of thought, hard work, and countless sleepless nights went into the making of this book. It was certainly not easy for us to make the Layers of Living Success plan. But we did it and it has helped countless people take control of their health. It has helped empower those who never thought Type 2 Diabetes could be reversed. It has helped me heal over one hundred patients (at the time of writing this)!

Mimi, and I poured our heart and soul into this project and we hope you love it. We absolutely love this program and have witness its success. We wish you health, happiness, and love!

Dr. Cheng Ruan

Made in the USA
Charleston, SC
22 October 2016